REFLECTIONS
OF A RELUCTANT
RETIREE

*Exercises to Inspire Us to Think About Living
a New Kind of Life in Our Later Years*

Richard G. Riedel

ISBN 978-1-63885-166-0 (Paperback)
ISBN 978-1-63885-180-6 (Digital)

Copyright © 2022 Richard G. Riedel
All rights reserved
First Edition

All rights reserved. No part of this publication may be reproduced, distributed, or transmitted in any form or by any means, including photocopying, recording, or other electronic or mechanical methods without the prior written permission of the publisher. For permission requests, solicit the publisher via the address below.

Covenant Books
11661 Hwy 707
Murrells Inlet, SC 29576
www.covenantbooks.com

PREFACE

Several years ago, I came across a devotional page in a book of daily meditations written by Frederick Buechner, a Presbyterian pastor, that he had entitled, *Listening to Your Life*. Initially he quoted the words of the Sports Columnist Red Smith who had this to say about writing:

> "Writing is really quite simple: all you have to do is to sit down at your typewriter and open a vein." "For my money," Buechner added, "the only books worth reading are books written in blood."

Then he added these words:

> "Write about what you really care about, is what he was saying. Write about what truly matters to you, not just things to catch the eye of the world but things to touch the quick of the world the way they have touched you to the quick, which is why you are writing about them. Write not just with wit and eloquence and style and relevance, but with passion. Then the things that your books make happen will be things worth happening. Things that make the people read them a little more passionate themselves for their pains, by which I mean a little more alive, a little wiser, a little more beautiful, a little more open and understanding. In short, a little more

> human. I believe that those are the best things that books can make happen to people, and we could all make a list of the particular books that have made them happen to us."

Since I had too much time on my hands and had given up the responsibility of putting a weekly Sunday message on paper, I thought I would sit down and put in print the thoughts that came my way as I read one book and another.

However, a funny thing happened on the way to the completion of my intended task. Well, maybe it was not so funny after all. The word *fortuitous* comes to mind. It happened while I was investigating the possibility of writing the words that follow: My doctor discovered a change in my EKG. Further examination and a heart catheterization later, I was on the operating table, having five bypasses surgically created that they said "would lengthen my life." The question that I asked myself was, *Why? Why did this happen to me?*

How come the blockages were discovered? By chance? Well, doctors tell me that I would have never made it to the hospital if a heart attack would have insinuated itself on my life. I would have died then and there, probably on the spot. So why? It was not to verify or prove the value of modern-day medical procedures and equipment. They are a common everyday experience. It was not to allow someone to practice their craft. There are many people to practice medicine on these days. The word *catheterization* is not even in the dictionary that has been on my desk for fifty plus years. So why?

I will be bold to say, "Because I have something more to do with my life." Now that is a rather presumptive statement to say the least. Yet I felt that I had some words to share, some thoughts to get out of my system. Words about starting over in one's later years after retirement. In any event, that is what happened and why I determined to keep on keeping on, putting on paper my thoughts about starting over again in one's life walk.

Certainly, everyone has some thought to share. Some do and some don't. I decided that I was someone who would do it.

Interestingly enough, I was reading another of Buechner's writings at the time of the event. So as I was in the process of coming out of the shadows of my surgery, I continued my interrupted reading of his book, *Secrets in the Dark*. The first chapter that I read, following my walk through the darkness, was one entitled, "A Room Called Remember!" Of course, it was a selection that talked about memories. This is what he writes:

> "We are all such escape artists, you and I. We don't like to get too serious about things, especially about ourselves. When we are with people, we are apt to talk about almost anything under the sun, except for what really matters to us, except for what is going on inside our own skins. We pass the time of day. We chatter. We hold each other at bay, keep our distance from each other, even when God knows it is precisely each other that we desperately need."

His suggestion is, I think that we are constantly in a state of trying to escape who we are—to escape, to forget our past. Then he suggests:

> There is a need within all of us, to enter the still room within us where the past lives on as part of the present, where the dead are alive again, where we are most alive ourselves, to the long journeys of our lives with all their twisting and turnings and to where our journeys have brought us. *The name of the room is Remember—the room where, with patience, with charity, with quietness of heart, we remember consciously to remember the lives that we have lived.* (Italics mine)

Later he adds this thought, "Hope stands up to its knees in the past and keeps its eyes on the future." And then concludes: "The past and the future. Memory and expectation! Remember and hope. Remember and wait. Wait for him, whose face we all of us know, because somewhere in the past we have faintly seen it, whose life we all of us thirst for because somewhere in the past we have seen it lived, have maybe even had moments of living it ourselves."

So in the after moments of that lifesaving experience—in these days when I seemed to be living beyond when I should have perhaps died—I took what I have learned in the past and reflect in that history on what I read in the present, hoping that I can speak to someone in a future time about all the possibilities that stand before them as they stood before me. Then it will be their turn...or maybe your turn!

ONE

It's Important to Have a Real Purpose in Your Life!

Retirement has both its good and its bad attributes. One of the really positive benefits is found in the fact that it affords an individual the opportunity to start over in life. It provides them with the chance to move out in a new direction or directions. It establishes the opportunity to fulfill some old possibilities and aspirations—more often than not—freed from the bindings of time, and the need to provide for one's family financial needs. At this point in one's life, they can make some fresh resolutions and open up a new door or two into a future that will have many clean, new, and unused opportunities. Yes, we can spell retirement: O-P-P-O-R-T-U-N-I-T-Y!

How many times during our "first life" were we confronted by a hope or a dream that had to be laid aside as we made our way through the demanding responsibilities of a life lived in the present tense? Bound by our family responsibilities and vocational demands, we put these seemingly idealistic dreams and aspirations in the back of our life's drawer, presuming that we would one day open it up and withdraw them and consider their accomplishment. Now, with a new life opening up before us, we have the chance to do just that. For the first time, we can consider those old but now new possibilities, and ponder their accomplishment. We can spell out the fulfillment of these hopes and dreams with these letters: S-A-T-I-S-F-A-C-T-I-O-N!

These opportunities can be either or both: visible and/or invisible. Some can be sought out and fulfilled in the world around us. Others can be accomplished in the world that is within us. Those we choose to engage in, in the world around us, will be open to the scrutiny and standards of others. Those we choose to satisfy inwardly will be judged by the standards we set for ourselves. Satisfaction can be gained in either or in both ways.

In the course of my years, I came across a book written by Louis L'Amour entitled, *Education of A Wandering Man*. It contained a recounting of the early years of L'Amour's life, what he read, and what he did. The book concluded with a list of readings he had accomplished over a seven-year period. Quite a list. What an education! One goal to be accomplished in life number two might be to read through all the books that one has encountered in life that were never read. We wished we had read the works of one author or another, but we passed them by. We told ourselves we just didn't have the time to read them. Maybe we didn't, but what better time to start and do that relished reading than now—today?

Roy Burkhart suggests that "if we set ourselves goals that can be grasped, how can the grasping be significant to us?" A reasonable thought, I believe; but then, how does one set a goal that is beyond one's grasp? I guess that the answer can be found in the word *aspiration*. My dictionary defines *aspiration* as a "lofty or ambitious desire." In other words, at this particular time in my life with the western boundary of my life span relatively close and a majority of my days lived out, other than my desire to give support, love, and encouragement to the members of my family, to what do I want to dedicate my life?

What goal or goals can I set for myself that I can seek to accomplish during the remaining days of my life? How am I going to spend my time for the rest of my life?

As Shakespeare might say, "That is the question!" It is one worthy of our consideration before it's too late.

Two

It is Important to Think about the End Before You Start at the Beginning!

During the days of the Black Revolution, at the conclusion of the second march from Selma to Montgomery, Alabama, Dr. Martin Luther King Jr. offered up this significant thought as he addressed those who marched with him or supported him:

> "It is not important how long the journey is. What is important is that we finish it. If you have the belief that you will finish it, that, in itself, makes the journey worthwhile."

In those words, Dr. King reminded me of some lines in a play by Joseph Ervine, *The Ship*. In the midst of that play, one of his characters—an old Mrs. Thurlow—is heard to say, "To me, the most wonderful thing in the world is not the young man beginning life with ideals, we all see that, but the old man dying with them undiminished." Always, both men were saying, "The journey continues."

I chanced to recall the life of a man I once knew. He started his vocational life on a farm. Later, as his horizon broadened, he ran for and was elected to a position in county government where he served for many years. As his age began to catch up with him, he completed his current term in office and began to use his accumulated interests and abilities to repair properties that he had come to own. I remember the time he fell through the floor of a porch on which he was working. He broke a number of bones. It hardly stopped him. Here was a man with a vision. His vision was to keep reinventing himself and to keep on living an active life. As long as he lived, his aspirations—his ideals—never diminished in size.

In their book, *Success Built to Last,* Jerry Porras, Stewart Emery, and Mark Thompson offer up this thought:

> "It's important to start with the end in mind, but it could be a dead end if you're in such a hurry to set a goal for yourself or for the sake of others that you don't think it through to the end."

It is important, therefore, when you set a goal, to begin with the end in mind!

"The goal-achieving process is both powerful and dangerous because it can make you effective at achieving objectives—to take a hill, as they say—without any assurance that it's the right mountain for you to climb. Goals don't come with a built-in guarantee that you'll benefit by reaching them or enjoy the process of getting there, nor do they assure you that you're on the right track. Goals, by nature, don't necessarily require focusing on inspiration as much as they do on perspiration and the sheer pragmatic effort of getting things done." The authors conclude this section with the question, "What are the important things worth doing with the time you have left?"

Somewhere out there, we have some idea or dream that needs to be envisioned and satisfied. We all have some inclination, but how many of us find ourselves in what Debbie Ford calls a "No-Cookie Zone?" (A No-Cookie Zone, according to Ms. Ford, is "often disguised, harmless choices that we create that keep us from spending our time doing something that will help us to accomplish some dream or aspiration that stands in the forefront of our mind's eye.") Our NCZs act like termites, eating away at the very foundation of our greatest life."

Our journey continues, but at the present moment, how many of us find ourselves spending time at a rest stop, wondering about the direction we need to take? What new adventures lie ahead of us? What should we do to add zest and enjoyment to the remaining years of our lives?

How about it?

THREE

It is Important to Find Opportunities to Make Changes in Your Life!

In one of his many books of sermons, Dr. James W. Moore, a Methodist minister serving a congregation in Houston, Texas, writes about dreams (I chose to call them *aspirations*). In his words, "When you lose your dream, you die. We have so many people walking around who are dead, and they don't even know it." Then he adds, "Anybody can grow older. That doesn't take any talent or ability. The idea is to grow up by finding the opportunity to change." And then he pens his final thought, "It's never too late to be all you can possibly be!"

Our concern in these pages is to find a new dream or two as we enter into the second stage of our lives. You have satisfied your initial vocational goal! You have had a part in creating a family and, probably, have also satisfied one hobby or another. I take the phrase, "It's never too late to be all you can possibly be," to mean that the abilities that I had at birth, and that were developed during my years of growing to maturity, now have the chance to be reborn and used in a new venue or dream.

In his book, *The Seven Habits of Highly Effective People*, Stephen Covey invites us to get involved in an interesting exercise. He asks us to imagine ourselves walking into a funeral parlor. You smell the flowers and hear the organ music. You walk down the aisle. You see the faces of people sitting in chairs, usually in a circle, and they're all people that you know, including the ones you love the most.

Everyone has a look of reverence on his or her face, a look of appreciation, and a look of sadness as well. You're not quite sure why they're there. You walk to the front of the room and see a casket. Looking into the casket, you come face-to-face with yourself. You are at your own funeral.

He conjectures, "Who will be the four people that have been invited to speak?" A family member, a colleague from work, a friend, someone from your civic circle? What kind of friend were you? What kind of parent were you? What kind of sister? What kind of coworker? What kind of neighbor were you? He finishes the section with these words, "Begin with the end in mind!" We have come across that phrase before.

I chanced upon this illustration again in the writing of another. This individual, upon reading this exercise, confessed to himself that "he was living his life in the 'right now' and wasn't—he suddenly realized—wasn't into leaving a legacy." He concludes his reflections with these words: "Ever since reading Covey's book, every important decision I've made has been based on one question: 'How do I want to be remembered?' Today I am literally writing my own eulogy with the way that I live my life. Of course, I am not perfect. I've fallen short on many things, but I can honestly say I have no regrets. If God took me home tonight, I would leave here dancing."

Maybe today is the day when we should start living our lives with the end in mind.

How do I want to be remembered? Do I want to go out with my boots on? How? When? Where?

We are in the process, whether we realize it or not, of writing our own life story. Word by word, sentence by sentence, paragraph by paragraph, chapter by chapter. We are succeeding or failing by the activities we have planned and by the commitments we have made. There is a dream that we were meant to satisfy. Do we know what it is? Friend, we don't want to die before we have seen that dream to completion. Do we?

It is still not too late!

Four

The Importance of a Few Extraordinary Choices!

Presuming that there is a possibility that each one of us can make a fresh start in our lives, no matter what our age or the time or place, then these words of Debbie Ford can be very helpful:

> "If we are willing to begin making a series of extraordinary choices now, we can turn the possibility of living our best life into a reality. All we need to do is begin by making a few choices each day."

I don't think that she means a whole lot of choices; rather, she means, there is a need to make a decision or two today that will enable us to point ourselves in some new direction or in several new directions, and make it or them a reality in our lives. The choices are—have to be made one at a time.

The question is, or the questions are: "What are the choices that one needs to make?" "What are the decisions that I must make?" "Can *I* make them?" "How do I search them out?" These are the questions that one might need a lifetime to answer. The problem is, we don't have a lifetime. We have only a few brief years, maybe fewer years than we imagine, left. Choices! Choices! Choices! How do I ferret them out in order that I can make one or a few extraordinary choices that will enable me to point my life in the right direction? I wonder.

I came across a book on a "sale table" in the bookstore that I frequent almost weekly. Written together by a husband and wife and entitled, *Live What You Love*—its introduction captured my attention. In reflection, they ask, "When did your dreams get buried under the responsibilities of adulthood? You reach a moment in time when you sense that something in your life needs to be changed, but you're too busy to stop and think about what it is. Now, today, you long for those almost-forgotten times when each day's accomplishments filled you with joy and excitement, when you embraced life with energy and enthusiasm. When there were a million special days."

The years of our lives pass, and the authors pay attention to that fact or problem and say of our present moments, "Now you sometimes feel as if you're stuck in a great big rut and, as the years go by, the rut keeps getting deeper and deeper. You sense loss, understanding that you were meant to do more. Now your dreams feel so far away and always seem to be just out of reach." Way out there; either in a yesterday or in a tomorrow that may never come, but always, always, they seem to be just out of reach.

Then the challenge: "Wouldn't it be awful to live your whole life and then say, 'Wait! I need another change. I just wanted to try this one thing.'" Finally, this observation: "Remember how scared you were to take the training wheels off your bike? Or how much courage it took for that first kiss? Nothing stopped you then. So what is stopping you now?"

Rethink Debbie Ford's thought: "If we are willing to begin making a series of extraordinary choices now, we can turn the possibility of living our best life into a reality." Time passes quickly, but our dreams remain. Some of them will take a significant amount of time to accomplish. The problem is, we have only so much of it left. Today, it might offer us our last best opportunity to begin to satisfy that dream or dreams that inhabit our minds, and tomorrow might be too late for us to say, "Wait! I need another change! I just wanted to try this one thing."

Today is the day to begin to try. Today is the day to begin again. So do whatever you are dreaming about today, or at least begin the journey toward the fulfillment of that dream.

Five

It All Comes Down to Taking Action!

When anyone sets out to change their style of living, they will inevitably encounter the warning of the pessimist and the wisdom of the shortsighted! "Be satisfied with what you have!" "The grass is not always greener on the other side of the fence!" "Be happy with what you have!" "Sit back and enjoy. You have earned the rest!" Those temptations are forever present. I, however, for one, am not satisfied with any one of them.

I have often thought about changing my environment and circumstance. I have made innumerable resolutions over the years, set some goals for myself, and assumed that I could change my life merely by saying, "I am going to do this or that!" Too often, however, I have failed to do what I said I was going to do and found myself lapsing back into my former ways of thinking and doing things. I have periodically and regularly closed the book on change.

So now, in this, the latter third of my life, when I find myself free of some of life's early encumbrances—like earning a living and helping to raise our kids—I ponder how I might change my direction and make a choice or two that I hope will be "lasting choices." I want to find a new challenge or two that will occupy my mind and body in this, hopefully, new-and-productive time in my life. So I find myself, once more, circling the wagons—to use a Texas term—to find a few protected peaceful moments where I can think through where I want to go and how I want to get there. I move round and round, looking for a new target—a new goal toward which I can point my life.

A sign reads, "To reach our goals we must, at times, run with the wind and, at times, against it!" Certainly, however, we must never stand still. It all comes down to taking action! Action is the accelerator. Taking focused actions that move us toward our goals and visions (aspirations) could be compared to being inside a finely tuned sports car, map in hand, ready to step on the gas.

John Nesbitt, in the writing that he entitled, *Mindset*, offers us this thought: "Many success stories are about men and women in their thirties or younger. But there is no age limit for a fresh start, adding experience to abilities. Sometimes such a new beginning starts with an end, taking a little shove to make a decisive step."

These words of George Bernard Shaw came to my attention, "The reasonable man adapts himself to the conditions that surround him. The unreasonable man adapts surrounding conditions to himself. All progress depends on the unreasonable man."

And then these words: "People are blaming their circumstances for what they are. I do not believe in circumstances. The people who get on in this world are the people who get up and look for the circumstances they want, and if they don't find them, they create them."

I have the fear of stepping on the accelerator! I know what I want to do. I know the direction in which I want to travel, but I just can't seem to push down on the pedal and proceed in the direction I want to go. So another day passes. I ponder my areas of interest and concern; the one's out there on the horizon, but I just can't seem to push the pedal down. Fear of failure? Uncertainty about the future? Maybe I will tomorrow? But will tomorrow come?

Friend, I have decided that today is the day to begin a new journey before I forget about what I want to do with the rest of my life. Tomorrow, here I come!

Six

We Must All Find a Sense of Purpose for Our Lives!

I was reminded of this fascinating slice of dialogue from *Alice in Wonderland*:

> Alice (speaking to the cat): "Would you please tell me which way I ought to go from here?"
> Cat: "That depends a good deal on where you want to go."
> Alice: "Oh, I don't much care."
> Cat: "Then it doesn't really matter which way you go."
> Alice: "But I want to go somewhere."
> Cat: "Oh, you are sure to do that."

How many people drift through life with no sense of direction and miss finding its meaning, as far as they are concerned? They never find their purpose and finally come up empty-handed, frustrated, depressed, and ashamed. Too late; they discover they have missed the mark that was set for them.

There is a real sadness to be found in not arriving at our intended destination and not realizing that we have not gotten there until it is too late for us to get there. I am hopeful that I will not come to that end, ashamed because I never found my way, never grasped my sense of mission—my unique purpose. If one knows their purpose, it makes life meaningful and zestful and joyous.

Yes, I am in search of that sense of purpose that will enable me to live out the remaining years of my life in a joyous mode. Debbie Ford writes: "When we feel good about ourselves, we give up our unrealistic expectations and stay grounded in reality. We draw healthy boundaries and take on only what we are likely to accomplish. When we are being true to our intent and vision and of who we aspire to be, we take the time to get clear about what we want, and we create a plan and structure to make sure we won't get lost along the way." I am trying to do that. However, I am probably being overly careful. I don't want to find myself moving in the wrong direction, and I know I am only one or two steps away, in each and every moment, from doing that.

A chance to utilize my past and my present moments; that is my first goal or aspiration. But often we can get lost in our caution, and by the time we reach the end of a sentence, we don't know why we began to write it down in the first place. Short sentences! That's the ticket! Aspirations around which we can place our hands, holding them tight until we determine their intent and purpose for our lives: a series of thoughts that will allow us to create a vision we can live with and a life we can treasure forever…

Be cautious, but not too cautious. Get on with it. It's your life!

Seven

It Is All Right to Do Things in Your Own Way!

In his writing, *Spiritually Incorrect*, author Dan Wakefield speaks of what he calls "the arrogance of Alcoholics Anonymous!" He notes that members of AA look down their noses on any individual who deals with their addiction in a way other than that prescribed by AA: the twelve-step way. They call such individuals "dry drunks!"

I am reminded that while I was in high school, our basketball coach would not allow us to shoot our free throws in the same way we shot our jump shots. Today, this is a common practice. We had to shoot them underhanded. His law was, "If you cannot make twenty-two of twenty-five shots your way, you must shoot them my way." Even though our percentage was probably not any better shooting them his way. So who was right? I think of comparing the golf swing of Jack Nicklaus, who is said to have a picture-perfect swing with that of Arnold Palmer—whose swing is not one to be emulated by anyone. Palmer's dad, a golf pro and teacher, saw no problem with his son's swing because he was winning with it. The same is said of Jim Furyk today.

I was reading, at the same time I was reading Wakefield's book, Gordon Livingstone's writing, *Too Soon Old, Too Late Smart!* He was writing of raising kids and how parents have a tendency to impair the development of their children by making them do things in a particular way. His discovery: "We are not obedient people!"

And so we are not! I pray in my own way! I read my own way! I garden in my own way. I swing my golf clubs in my own way! I do a whole lot of things in my own way. I like Frank Sinatra's rendition, "I'll do it my way!" Granted, the ways of my parents sometime make an appearance, but I like doing things in my own way. I feel more comfortable doing it my way. Yes, I have some cultural and religious limits in what I do. I do have to be sure that what I am faring is correct in those sorts of ways, but after that, it's my ball game; so I can play it the way I want to.

I may not be right! I may not achieve the heights that others do. I do, however, get along, and in the end, well—what did the wise man say, "What does it profit a man if he gain the whole world and lose his own soul!" (Interpretation, my own!) I want to keep my soul and I want to get all I can out of the world in which I live, but I want to do it my way!

So I keep on trying to hone my habits by what I read and what I see others doing, but I do what I want to do, in my own way; and God willing, I will achieve something and be satisfied with it.

EIGHT

You Must Live Your Best Day Every Day!

In her writing, *The Best Year of Your Life*, Debbie Ford offers up this thought:

> "We must muster up the courage to go out and make the most of every day. We must take the time to listen to the cries of our own souls and have the faith to make changes and take risks. Excellence requires us to have the courage to live up to how we have lived our lives to this point and go after something that is totally unknown.
>
> "To live a life of excellence, you will have to take risks. You will have to step into new territory and climb new mountains. To leave your mark in the world, you will have to stand someplace you've never been willing to stand before. To create an extraordinary life, you will have to be present in each moment and give one hundred percent of yourself. You will have to commit each day to being the best you can be and aspire to perform your daily tasks in the most conscious way possible. Living your best requires you to take a moment each time you're about to make a decision or put something into your body, and

make sure that move reflects the very highest choice you can make. Aspiring to excellence is a commitment that you must make each day when you open your eyes."

Such a determination was hard, if not impossible, in your growing up and maturing years. To say it will be easy, today—in the follow-up years of your life with a majority of your time having now been put into your past—is to throw sand into the wind.

Remember the old expression, "You have to put your best foot forward. If you do your part, if you take one step forward expressing all the greatness that lives within you, the universe will take a hundred steps toward you."

These thoughts need to be underscored. We must muster up the courage to go out and make the most of every day. We will have to take risks! We will have to stand someplace we have never been willing to stand before and give a hundred percent of ourselves to perform our daily tasks in the most conscious way possible. So…

NINE

We Are All Created to Be Someone and to Do Something!

"Life is made up of changes. As we grow older, we do not function as well physically as we did in our youth. So the time to serve God is now." Amen and amen. The writer of these words, Stuart Briscoe, a Wisconsin pastor of a small mega church, concludes his words with this statement:

> "We shouldn't wait until we are old to be what we were created to be. Even though we are young, we are created to be someone and to do something. We need to get on with it…"

Okay, but what if you did something you wanted or thought you wanted to do, and now you are old and all of that is behind you?

This morning, as I channel-surfed my way through the television channels available to me, I came across an old film on the life—or most of the life—of the fame Supreme Court jurist, Oliver Wendell Holmes. He was a great mind and a great lover. The film speaks of his wonderful relationship with his wife as he journeyed through the positive and negative experiences of a justice on the nation's highest court.

The first concluding scene in the film presents to the viewer his retirement from the court. At the age of ninety, following a confusing morning on the bench, he packs up his robe and retires to his home. Another final theme comes on a later day. It shows him taking a walk on a piece of ground that separates the Washington Monument from the Lincoln Memorial. A little boy is flying a paper airplane that needs fixing. The retired jurist tells the boy that he can fix the plane. As he tries to do so, he comes across a headline on the paper that has been used to make the plane. It is an announcement of his retirement. He fixes the plane and gives it a human nudge, and it flies away. He then walks to the memorial.

One thing that came to mind as I thought about that scene is that life is fleeting, and though we may play a significant role in its ongoing development, time passes us by. Another is that we all have some time in the race that Holmes called "the cantor:" the slowdown time when we finish the race of life with a flurry.

Holmes's life lasted until he was well over ninety, and for most of those retirement years—sixty-five until ninety-plus—he was still engaged as a member of the Court, using a practical mind to serve his country. Those of us who are older can contradict Mr. Briscoe by saying, "We are enjoying the last of life for which the first was made." We are using it for our own and for the world's benefit! I wonder, can you say that? Really say that and mean it? Why?

TEN

We Can Do Things for Fun That We Used to Get Paid For!

This is an interesting thought. We need to give it some attention. "Retirement should not be about the ceasing of work, because people were created to be productive. Retirement should be a season in which a person has a new liberty to engage in a different kind of service. We should be honoring the Lord, benefiting society, and finding fulfillment until the day we die."

The man who wrote those words, he was not retired when he wrote them. Now I know that he is retired, I wonder if those words make sense to him now. I don't think the problem is *in* retiring: the problem is *about* retiring. The words, "Retirement should be a season in which a person has a new liberty to engage in different kinds of services." We have to ask ourselves, prior to our engagement or investment in them, "Are they worthy of our time and interest?" One question that arises as we look out at the world and ponder new occupations and directions: If we spent our entire life honing our gifts in one direction, is it possible to stop, go back to "go," and begin moving in another direction? I think that is possible. Maybe a little difficult, but possible nonetheless.

Somewhere, I read that a good manager can engage themselves in any kind of organization. In recent years, for example, several business types have been appointed to lead a number of our big-city school districts—Chicago and New York City being two of them.

Now I don't know how they did or are doing, or if they are still at it; but—well, the point I wish to make is, their management skills, their human relations gifts, and abilities could be well-adopted to a school situation. So their accumulated accomplishments and experience should be quite useful in such an endeavor. They seem to prove the validity of such a possibility.

In the long run, I choose to look at the above-quoted words as meaning we can enjoy doing something for fun that we used to get paid for doing! We can, on the other hand, reach out and take up the mantle of a new job as well, and strengthen our gifts by building up a new set of responsibilities. *Retirement* in this guise would be a life without the certain stress that we put aside when we retired. In this new vocational endeavor, we will, of course, assume another kind of stress because all situations produce their own brand of stress-related factors. However, the stress levels will not, very likely, be comparable nor life threatening.

All this, I buy, but with certain provisos. The second part of my life, which I am now living, demands that I impose some regular checkup times on my plans. I have to ask myself, at periodic intervals, if I am continuing to move in my anticipated direction? Is what I am doing continuing to be a practical and positive use of my time? Do I need to reassess my intentions and my goals?

Frankly, at this point in time, I am the only one who can truly evaluate my activities. It is my time and my life. I have only so much time to give to my family and to myself. I have to be sure that I am not cheating and ignoring them as I engage myself in one adventure or another.

I have moved, in my own lifetime, through three retirements. The last two jobs were more fun than work. Isn't that what retirement is all about? I am in the process of finding fulfillment every day, ofttimes in a new way. I know now that stress is a basic ingredient in the life of someone on the go, but let it come. I know that I can handle it. So I keep my eyes looking ahead of me and keep my life in an "active mode!"

Eleven

We Need to Consider What the Next Step in Our Life Is Going to Be

In his writing, *Too Soon Old, Too Late Smart*, Dr. Gordon Livingston writes:

> "All of life is a gamble in which we don't get to deal the cards, but are nevertheless obligated to play them to the best of our abilities."

A fact of life, "Do with it with what you have!" So most of us do. However, once you have done it with what you have, what do you have left over to do it (the retirement years) with? That, of course, is the question that I find myself struggling to answer. It is a question that we often seek to avoid because many of us really don't know what to do today, in our second lifetime, with what we have left.

What do I have left? What do I have left to deal with what is coming into my life?

History books, so someone has said, "seek to tell us about the past." Prognosticators are those people who take their knowledge of that history and then proceed to tell us what the future might hold in store for us. It is not about being clairvoyant. It is about being perceptive. It is about noticing what is around the corner.

Being forward-looking differentiates one group of people from another. It is a skill level that many of us do not possess, so we have to rely on others to suggest what the future holds in store for us and others like and around us. We are called upon to deal with the information that these other people lay out before us and, while we are living within its boundaries, create new things. One group of writers declare: "To leave something meaningful behind, we have to devote ourselves to creating something valuable ahead."

We receive a legacy from those who have gone before us. We leave a legacy to those who follow us. We have the opportunity to reference the past and, in the process, create a new future. We are to be different, to be new people! Constantly, therefore, we are to be in the process of finding new purposes for our lives. It is to reflect, and then—based upon those moments of self-inventory—invent or reinvent ourselves. The results become history, our history, and a part of the history of our descendants. We are to be constantly in a quest for newness.

In the time of passage, when we move from our necessary labors into those years when we are able to rest from our labors (we call this retirement), we need to be in a state of finding ourselves or refinding ourselves, seeking to find out who we are so we can determine what we will be. My retirement journey means that in addition to finding a new purpose for my life, I need to be involved in seeking to become the kind of person I want to be remembered by my family and those around me.

Although we will be remembered, at least our obituary might, in part, show who we were in our formative and growing-up years; our real legacy will be determined by what we do in the years that are lived after the gold watch is presented to us. In those times, we can become what we were finally intended to be. These are the years for which people will really remember us, as they look down at us for the last time—as they bid us farewell.

Maybe today becomes a time for a new beginning. Get it? Every day is the time for a new beginning, or as the philosopher said it, "The next step is the first step to the rest of your life." I am looking forward to being able to take that second step!

Twelve

We Are Not Alone in Our Quest for Life!

As I read my way through Gordon Livingston's book, *Too Soon Old, Too Soon Smart*, I came across this series of statements that summarize much of my thinking up to this point in my life. Let me share them with you:

> "Everything we are afraid to try, all of our unfulfilled dreams, constitute a limitation on what we are and what we could become."

> "So much of our lives consists of broken promises to ourselves."

> "We often do not do what is necessary to become the people we want to be."

> "The fear that we might try and not succeed can produce a crippling inertia. Keeping our expectations low protects us from disappointment."

> "Where do we find the determination and patience required to achieve the things we want?"

> "We have become used to the idea that much of what we don't like about ourselves and our lives can be quickly overcome with little effort on our part."

> "Alteration of our attitudes and behavior is a slow process: change is incremental."

These are all relatively true statements. They provide us with no answers, but the doctor provides us with a lot of wisdom for living. They don't say much more than I perhaps have written, but they tell me that I am not alone in my quest for something. I suspect that the one that speaks loads to me is this one: "The fear that we might try and not succeed can produce a crippling inertia. Keeping our expectations low protects us from being disappointed."

As I reread those words, I was in the process of reading another book entitled, *You've Got to Read This Book*. It is a series of essays written by individuals who found that their life was changed through an encounter with one book or another. The one that spoke to me was in the writing of John St. Augustine. The book, *Instant Replay: The Green Bay Diary of Jerry Kramer*. Since I have been a Packer fan all my life, it captured my attention. This is what St. Augustine wrote:

> "Reading *Instant Replay* allowed me to relive the 1967 championship season from beginning to end with the most successful team (on and off the field) in the history of the sport…I began to think that becoming the best I could be, should be the number-one-priority in my life, no matter what I decided to do. It was pretty powerful stuff for a ten-year-old."

And it was and is for someone much older.

These words of Packer coach Vince Lombardi look at me from my office wall: "Winning is not a sometime thing; it's an all-time thing. You don't win once in a while; you don't do things right once in a while; you do them right all the time. Winning is a habit. Unfortunately, so is losing."

So again, the message is, "Get on with it, friend!" Burn some bridges! Step out in front of yourself and follow your best thoughts. I wish I could. Oh, how I wish I could. The question is, Is that day in sight? Oh, how I hope it is.

We need to *do* what is necessary to become the people we want to be! Remember, "winning is an all-time thing!" Get on with it!

Thirteen

We Need an "Itch" to Get Us Going or Keep Us Going!

Some years ago, while attending a party in the suburbs of Pittsburgh, Pennsylvania, I was introduced to one of the local television personalities of the day. She and her dog were featured on one of the daily morning programs offered to the children in our home. She had a real enthusiasm on the air, one that was immediately contagious in whatever place she found herself. It was catching! We caught it that night! I was surprised when I met her. Her hair was already streaked with gray, probably something that was family related, because at that time, I think she was just in her mid-thirties.

Somehow in the conversation she was having with someone else, mention was made of her gray hair. Her response: "Yes, there is snow on the mountaintop, but believe me, there is a fire in my belly!" Today, all these years later and I am well past my mid-thirties, that is exactly how I feel. There *is* snow on the mountaintop; though I must admit, I don't know what is going on in my belly—physically speaking—because age does odd things to your insides. However, I really don't feel a day older than the day I left graduate school, though my wife would say that I nap a lot. Oh, I have a few other aches and pains, and I don't get in and out of my car as easily as I used to; but then, a two-seat car is hard to get into—always and for most everyone of my age. You just have to back your way in. Getting out has its problems too.

The point is, I seem to have a continuing itch to be doing something, to get going, to be going somewhere...

In the meantime—that is, between projects—I find myself seeking to prepare for whatever might dawn upon my horizon. I remember a print of a painting that hung on the wall in my fourth-grade classroom. In fact, I found it in many classrooms in my growing-up years. It pictured a young Abraham Lincoln cutting wood. He had stopped to rest. His axe was leaning against the base of a tree that he was cutting down. His foot rested on the top of some cut wood, and he had a book in his hand, which he was reading, during a rest period he had taken for himself. The caption below the picture read: "I will study and get ready for my time, which is soon to come."

It is said, historically speaking, that there was probably just one second in history in which the Soviet Union was willing to hand over East Germany to the West and NATO. It tells us—history, that is—that Helmut Kohl, the German chancellor, caught that moment. The important factors that played a role in his preparation for that moment were found in his repeated announcements that unification was going to happen and in his ability to initiate some practical steps to achieve the unification, including the use of his diplomatic contacts in Moscow and Washington. Many others couldn't have seized that historic moment the way Kohl did. Looking back, this is what he wrote:

> "When we began our walk to the unification in autumn of 1989, it was like the transition of a high moor. We stood in the water to our knees, fog hid the view, and we just knew there must be a path somewhere. We didn't know exactly where it was. Step-by-step we moved on and came quickly to the other side. Without the help of God, we wouldn't have made it."

Planning and preparation paid off again. It always does.

So in these years, walking in and between one project and another, I read and pray and exercise and anticipate and wonder,

What does the future hold in store for me? What does tomorrow *hold in store for me?* I know that I can't walk too far into the future at my age, but I can be ready for anything that the future might put in my path, might hold in store for me, today. I can, and so can you! Can't you?

Fourteen

There Is Always Time to Begin Again!

Just before a spring vacation break, a school bus driver issued new bus passes to each of his youthful riders, as they boarded the vehicle, and asked them to deposit their old, frazzled passes—one's they had been carrying since the start of the school year—in a basket near his seat. He said he wanted them to have new, clean, legible passes for his successor whom they would meet following the vacation period. He told those who asked him the why of it all: that he was going to spend the vacation time in Las Vegas. If he won, he was going to retire.

On the first day of school, following the vacation, that very same driver opened the bus door in silence, and as his young passengers boarded, he checked each new clean white card as if he had never seen it or the student before; and they responded in much the same way.

I am sure that most of us, given one situation or another, have thought about beginning our lives all over again. I don't mean moving to a new location or of moving from one job to another. I mean just that: starting out our lives all over again—returning to *go* and beginning again.

Well, that is the possibility that is available to us on the first day following our retirement. We can begin to walk in any direction we want to. Practically speaking, we can assess our possibilities and probabilities and utilize them to walk our lives in a new direction.

I read of an academic type who had always wanted to learn how to play the violin. As the time finally became available in his schedule, he began to take lessons; and after several years, he invited some friends who played orchestral instruments to join him in playing a recital for some other friends. Having accomplished his first dream, he decided to learn to speak French. He went to a local university and did just that. Subsequently, he invited some friends to a meal in his home, the only requirement being that they speak only French while they were at the table. I did not learn what he did after that.

The point is, consider the possibilities available to us to do things like that—to make our dreams a living reality in our lives. The opportunities are, realistically speaking, almost endless.

I chanced to see these words on a church bulletin board one afternoon: "Whatever your past has been, your future is spotless!" So pick up your life's pen and begin to write a new chapter in your life. And begin today!

FIFTEEN

It Is Forever Possible for Us to Rethink Our Past and Redirect Our Futures!

In her book, *When the Heart Waits*, Sue Monk Kidd tells of a conference she attended. During the event, each of the participants was given a sheet of colored paper and was asked to tear it into a shape that they felt represented their lives. While these were being collected—sometime later—and being used to create a large collage, someone else came around with a glass bowl to collect the scraps of paper that had been torn off and destined to be thrown away. The jar was then placed on an altar. The conference leaders said, "Only by gathering up this confetti of scars and torn pieces, only by embracing it and setting it on an altar can we begin to transform it."

    I am not sure what the intended results of this activity were, but the exercise did speak to me as I read of the incident. That is, while each of us—when asked to talk about the "high spots" in our lives—are prone to speak only of positive, successful, and heartwarming events, I wondered if there is not a place in such discussions to think of the negatives; those not-so-successful situations and events that also have been present in our lives and their development? When we are assessing our lives and telling our life's story to ourselves and others, well, someone has written: "We need to go boldly down into our not-so-positive experiences through therapy, art, journaling, active imagination, and bodywork, etc., and spend some time mucking around and getting to know our lives in their entirety."

"It's common sense," writes Annie Dillard, "that when you move in, you try to learn the neighborhood."

So it would seem at various junctures in our lives—as we look at the neighborhood we have built through our experiences, relationships, and the like—for us to look at *all* that, is part of our adventure, even those situations and events that we might like to forget; for each one of them also plays a role in the person we have become.

There is a time and place, in other words, when we need to see the whole of our lives as one complete accumulation of events to see how one event or relationship might have had an impact on another. How many situations and experiences have and continue to impact on who we are and what we do today? If we were to catalogue each of these situations, experiences, and relationships, might they not assist us in handling and/or speaking to those we relate to and will continue to communicate with in both the present and future moments of our lives?

There is so much to be learned, and maybe more, from the scraps of our lives that we have tended to forget and push out of our memories. We need to possess, as best we can, the whole of our life's story. The forgotten events may and will continue to play a sometimes silent role in all that we say and do today. We need to be aware of them. Maybe our children need to know all about the journeys we have taken, even the ones that we would like to forget, for they are the result of both the negative and positive events in our lives.

Harold Kushner, in his writing, *Overcoming Life's Disappointments*, suggests that sometime after Moses came down from the Sinai Mountain with the second set of tablets containing the Ten Commandments (you will remember that, in a fit of anger, he threw the original Decalogue to the ground, breaking the stones into many pieces), that he stopped and stooped down and gathered up the pieces of the original tablets and placed them along with the new ones in the Ark of the Covenant. He says that, maybe, "They will tell us that the Covenant has been broken, but that it can be renewed, [that] the covenant relationship between God and his people has been damaged but not ended."

He then asks this question, "What does a person do with all the dreams that don't come true, dreams of wealth and recognition, dreams of marriage and family?" His answer, "True success consists not in becoming the person you dreamed of being when you were young, but in becoming the person you were meant to be, the person you are capable of being, when you are at your best."

It is important to discuss our whole life with our descendants and encourage them to ask *the right questions* in order that we might share with them the answers to who we are and what they may become.

Sixteen

It Is Important to Have a Sense of Direction in Your Life!

How many times have we heard it? Our son or daughter, or a son or a daughter of a friend is living at home; or he or she is going back to school! Why? The inevitable answer: "To find themselves." One cynical parent suggested that in the course of an especially prolonged search, his child had had time to find several people.

Dr. Gordon Livingston, in his writing, *Too Soon Old, Too Late Smart*, notes:

> "Though a straight line appears to be the shortest distance between two points, life has a way of confounding geometry. Often it is the dalliances and the detours that define us. There are no maps to guide us on our most important searches. Rather, we must rely on hope, chance, intuition, and a willingness to be surprised."

A *dalliance* is a pause we make in life *because* we don't know where we are, and we certainly don't know where we are going. A *detour* is a dalliance gone wrong. Now I am not sure where I am, but wherever it is, many have been here or there before me. Furthermore, many more will be there tomorrow or are there today. I kind of know where I have been, so I think I know where I am; but as to where I want to go, that puts us into a situation we might call a dalliance.

I certainly don't want to start out on a journey in the wrong direction. At this point in my life, I don't have the time for that. Careers are sometimes made up of detours, but I don't have time for a new career. I only have time for a short journey, so I am using the present moments as a dalliance. I am standing with one foot fixed to make a new step but unwilling to stretch it out and place it on the ground in one direction or another because I don't want to make a false step. So caught in the grip of (is it fear?), I stand in one place, wishing to go forward but unable to decide when or why I should begin a new journey. How many people are like that? What about *you*?

It is easy to say, "I want to be surprised!" As I write those words, I wonder to myself, *Do I believe that?* Upon further reflection, I must say, "I don't think so!" I think I want to be convicted as to where I want to go and how I am going to get there. It is too late for surprises!

I could offer up the prayer, "Lead, Lord, and thy servant will follow." The answer would, of course, be a surprise! I am afraid of such an affirmation or prayer. It speaks of an open road and an unchartered destination. Surprise! Surprise! Do I need a sign, or to hear a voice that says to me, *Go in this direction*, or *Go in that direction*? Am I waiting for that voice?

Frankly, my experience in life tells me that I will never hear that voice because my life is waiting for me to make a decision and follow it! So I have the choice of dilly-dallying in the time and place where I am, or making a calculated determination to step out in a direction of my own choosing, and come what may, following it to its conclusion.

Like it or not, that is the only choice before me! I have got to decide what I am going to do with the rest of my life; and I had better decide quickly, or life will make the decision for me. The result of that act of indecision? Surprise! Surprise!

So today, or not later than tomorrow, this is my decision, and this is my plan to carry it out…

Seventeen

It Is Important to Be Ready to Allow Change to Take Place in Our Lives!

I don't know how many farmers still sow their seed by hand, broadcast style. The answer is probably *none*! At least I haven't seen any doing it in my lifetime. However, since I am not a farmer nor a gardener of any note (who knows?), my only experience with "broadcasting" is the organized kind. I lay out some strips of flowers, using one of those packages available in the seed department of a store. I put it in an area of our yard, put some dirt over it, and begin to water it regularly. Then I wait for the seeds to grow.

As I remember it, the last time I did it, I never saw the anticipated flowers. I must admit, however, that the problem was probably with me and not with the manufacturer. I am more familiar with the dig-the-hole, push-in-the-seed, replace-the-dirt kind of planting procedure.

I was thinking of the whole philosophy of planting—if one can call it a philosophy from a vocational point of view—this morning. I am looking for something to do. I need to find a place where I can invest the rest of my life. I am the seed, and I need a place where I can plant myself for the benefit of myself and the worlds in which I live.

Looking at my options, at the many possible places where I could plant myself in the hopes that I might grow into something valuable and/or useful, the thought of broadcasting myself does not seem like a reasonable way to go. To cast my bread upon the waters of the vocational landscape is rather risky, considering my age. Seed (myself) in hand, I am looking for a place where I can plant myself the old-fashioned way with some real, personal effort.

I am qualified physically but not mentally to be a greeter in a Walmart Store. I am, to quote some members of my family, "too technologically challenged" to work in a computer store. I would be dangerous at Lowe's or Home Depot! My areas of interest would negate the possibility of my working in a Barnes & Noble or Borders Bookstore, though that is a possibility. I know I am not ready for a rocking chair or a daily walk in the park.

I knew a doctor who was a brilliant diagnostician. He could spot the reason for a child's ailments immediately. Sadly, he had to retire from the practice of medicine because he lost most of his sight; he was judged "legally blind." He would have been great in an office, seeing children, and making recommendations to another doctor concerning treatment and medication. However, the malpractice insurance rate was too high for any doctor to take him on, or maybe it would have created some professional jealousy; so he spent the final years of his life at home, lonely and frustrated.

There are many fields today that advertise for and encourage men and women to reenter the marketplace. There are others that see older people as a deterrent to the professional development of those who are younger. Many in the younger generations see older and experienced individuals as rivals. They don't have the same work ethic: too many of those old folk lived to work; many of their younger successors work to live! They could not countenance their presence in their workplace. So as we see people living longer, more vital lives, we have a whole cadre of workers feeling like the world has passed them by, even though they have so much to offer to that world.

The question of what we are to do, I mean retired folks like myself, baffles us. We need to be on the offensive, but we are not sure of our goals or possibilities. As you can sense, I have no answers, just questions.

Someone wrote, and their words came to my attention, "Sow your seed. Have realistic expectations!" A voice says to me, *Try some-*

thing new! Where? The voice hasn't answered that question for me as of yet. "Try something new"?

I remember reading that Louis Pasteur, the same guy who discovered that most infectious diseases are caused by germs and, with his work, laid the foundation for what today we call microbiology, said: "Change favors the prepared mind. I was ready!"

I, too, am ready. I just don't know what I am ready for. So today I wonder what the future might hold in store for me. I will keep looking for an answer.

I keep these words on the computer screen before me. Sow your seed! Have realistic expectations! Sow your seed! Have realistic expectations! Sow your seed! Have realistic expectations! Sow your seed…

I can do nothing else or more. I can only, in the words of the Boy Scout motto, "Be prepared," and wait and keep looking… I am looking! I continue to wait!

EIGHTEEN

You Have an Opportunity to Leave a Legacy!

In the introduction to their book, *A Leader's Legacy*, James Kouzes and Barry Posner offer a series of propositions worthy of our consideration. They begin, "The legacy you leave is the life you lead!" It was a title they thought they would give to their book that was finally entitled *A Leader's Legacy*.

In the book, they offer us these suggestions: "Thinking about a legacy can be extremely energizing and uplifting. It forces us to think about today's actions in a larger context." Then this statement, "The legacy perspective explicitly reveals that we make a difference. Then the only question remaining to consider is, what kind of a difference do I want to make?" A heartfelt quest to leave a lasting legacy is a journey from success to significance.

They got down to deeper business with this declaration: "Legacy-thinking means dedicating ourselves to making a difference, not just working to achieve fame and fortune. It also means appreciating that others will inherit what we leave behind."

This exercise follows: "By asking ourselves how we want to be remembered, we plant the seeds for living our lives as if we matter. By living each day as if we matter, we offer up our own unique legacy. By offering up our own unique legacy, we make the world we inhabit a better place than we found it."

How do I want my kids to remember me? What accomplishments do I want to be remembered for? Have I accomplished all that

I was intended to do; or at this point in time, as I think back over my life, are there some holes that need plugging, some dreams that need fulfillment, and some hopes that need satisfaction?

Maybe after all is said and done, I have not really satisfied my hopes and dreams, and I need to redirect my efforts so that I can leave behind me something of which I and those who follow me can always be proud of.

It's reflection time! Ready! Set! Think! Do!

Nineteen

You Need to Use All the Time That You Are Given!

A business type declares, "I got up, and putting first things first, I read the *Wall Street Journal*, the *New York Times*, and the *Washington Post*. Then I had breakfast." Give me a break! The *Princeton Packet* and the *Times* or the *Post* or the *Journal*; but all three? Come on! I read of a Texas minister who said that he read the Sunday Morning *New York Times* before he shaved and showered, had breakfast, and went to the church he served to conduct several morning worship services. I don't think so! Maybe, "I skimmed some of the sections of the *Times*, and then I had breakfast," but…

A recent issue of a business journal speaks about how successful people conduct their workdays. You know, up at 5:30 a.m. and home at 8:30 p.m. One of the men followed, supposedly, gets up daily at 3:30 a.m. and doesn't get home until 10:30 p.m., when he kisses his wife goodnight. First mention that he had a wife. A second has a girlfriend, and the third is single. So much for successful and happy living. How many wives or girlfriends? How many children? No mention is made of them in any story. How many separations or divorces? Is that successful, happy living? How does one define success? How long does success last? How many of these individuals, in a short period of time, fall into the land of oblivion? All day, every day from 3:30 a.m. until 10:30 p.m.? It's hard to believe. I must admit, I am remarkably impressed by such a work ethic or habit.

All my life I tried to figure out how to discipline myself and to get the most done in the least amount of time so I could have a life. I read countless numbers of books, attended any number of seminars, whatever; but here I am, some fifty years later, wondering how to do it. So I continue to read magazines, like the one mentioned above, and books, and the question remains, "How do I do everything I need to do, and still have time for what I want to do if what I want to do is more than do my job?"

Then I remembered some words I read before I began my quest. "Very early the next morning, long before day, Jesus got up and left the house. He went out of town to a lonely place, and there, he prayed." That is from the New Testament, Book of Mark.

Then I reread some information in the article mentioned above. It said, on separate pages, "Give yourself a time-out!" "Devote an hour to uninterrupted thinking and planning every day." "The first thing in the morning is the safest. Use that time to think *strategically* about your work."

And this paragraph by another writer: "Fight for your right to think. Declare the first hour of every workday email free. There is nothing that cannot wait fifty-nine minutes in your box!

Remember, there are two thousand years separating the first note and the second recommendation. How much money could I have saved? How many hours could I have devoted to something else? I am still searching and thinking and trying... I think there is still hope for me. How are you doing?

Someone has written, "Jesus repeatedly teaches that it is not how much time we have that counts, but what we do with the time we have." The commodity here is time! An old lesson is still good if we follow it! Right?

Twenty

Every Discipline Has at Least One Purpose!

Here is another tidbit from the writing of Dr. Gordon Livingston's book, *Too Soon Old, Too Late Smart*: "We are not obedient people!" He reminds us, if we need the reminding, that "self-discipline is something that many of us find impossible to effect in our lives." Let me add another thought to his, "One of the things that defines us is what we worry about!"

I have a discipline, and I worry, in a sense, whenever a day passes by and I do not effect it in my life. It is a reading discipline. I do it in order that I might feel a sense of accomplishment every day. It is not an overwhelming discipline. I read maybe from four or five books, plus some passages from a study Bible, and an article or two in one magazine or another. I do it, mostly, as mentioned above because it gives me a sense of accomplishment and fulfillment each day. "I have not lived today in vain!"

Later on, Livingston writes: "Fear, while effective in the short term, is not useful in producing lasting change. The use of it as a motivator for behavior ignores the fact that there are no more powerful desires than the pursuit of happiness and the struggle for self-respect."

Spiritually speaking, St. Augustine speaks to the situation with his quotable statement: "Our hearts are restless until they find themselves in thee (God!)." I think he meant that God has given us some internal directives which we have to decipher and learn for ourselves.

Nobody else can do it for us. We have to do it by ourselves. Our ultimate quest is to find ourselves, for in doing so, we find ourselves; and in the process, we also find happiness and a sense of self-respect.

It relates to what I have been thinking about all along. We need a pattern to guide us through the retirement years of our lives. We need something to help us gauge how successful we are in our waking hours. I guess that is why Livingston notes that fear is the impetus for us to do something. Let me call it a "desire for self-worth and for a sense of accomplishment."

What is it that causes our wheels to turn? It is one thing for me, and another thing for you. However, whatever it is in the long run, it is finding a sense of satisfaction and completion, making the accomplishment of those two desires an important part of each of our days. That will enable us to do what we want to do during the remainder of each day. "A discipline a day keeps a feeling of emptiness away."

Another Livingston quote: "If it is true that no one on their deathbed wishes that they had spent more time in the office, what does that suggest for directing our efforts?" One needs to find satisfaction in their work or in their avocations: they need to discover a sense of fulfillment that will enable them to go to sleep each night *peacefully*! So what is the discipline that, once established, will enable *you* to enjoy the living out of each one of *your* days?

Twenty-One

We Need to Remind Ourselves That Every Day Is Special!

In his writing, *Spiritually Incorrect*, Dan Wakefield speaks of the positive attitude evidenced by a former Miami Dolphins football player, Jim Mandich, almost every day of his life. Evidently, Mandich, when asked how he felt or was feeling, on most occasions, was always very positive in his responses. One of his standard rejoinders struck a chord with me: "Every day's a holiday, and every meal's a banquet!"

What did this say to me? This! Every day is special! Every event has something to give me! As an individual in retirement or in the second half of life, to use a term attributed to Bob Buford, there is something uplifting in those words. I thought yesterday of spending some time at the end of each day, reflecting on the events that had transpired as I lived through it. Today I thought about the fact that one should also begin each day with a plan or sense of optimism.

On the major patriotic holidays, Memorial Day and July Fourth, I would awaken, as a child, with the thought, *We are going to a parade today!* Later we would meet my grandparents on the lawn of the city hall, in the town in which I grew up, and together we would watch a parade. It seemed like everyone in town was there, either in the parade or watching it, adults and kids alike. The sidewalks and streets were always overflowing with people. We, however, always stood on the city hall lawn. It was a great place to meet and find one another. There was also a water fountain close by (we used to call it "a bubbler") so we could refresh ourselves if the parade was late in starting. It was a wonderful vantage point from which to watch the activities on the street before us. It was a very special day, and the day went uphill all the way, beginning with the parade and ending with the fifty-cent piece that my grandfather would always give me. What a deal! Watch a parade and get paid for doing so! Wow!

Every day *ought* to have a purpose, and once the purpose is discovered, planned for, and then implemented, it cannot help but be a holiday. So, too, if there is a purpose, there is also a goal to be reached; and in moments of reflection, once it has happened and its activities have been accomplished, one can take satisfaction in a job, hopefully, well-done. And not only that, for always there is the possibility that there will be some spill over into tomorrow. That, however, is a goal to be incorporated into a new day. "Every day is a holiday!"

"Every meal is a banquet!" One of the purposes of these personal reflections is, "What lesson did I garner from today's reading?" That is, in addition to whatever new things I have learned, what lesson did I receive? I am always amazed at all that races through my mind when I find a phrase or a sentence or paragraph that stimulates my thought processes. Things of my past come to mind and meet me in the present moments of my today. Things of the present seem to be magnified by that surge of thoughts that arise, as they come from my past into the present moment. Suddenly, tomorrow takes on some new possibilities. Every day is special because of the ingredients it places on my table. I just have to check them in the evening.

I can still find the rewards of satisfactions past today, and then I can begin to find some new feelings of accomplishment as I place some of today's decisions and happenings beside them.

"Every day's a holiday, and every meal's a banquet!" They sure are…

Twenty-Two

We Need to See How Important It Is to Mend Our Mistakes!

Someone, after reading through the biblical account of Jesus's feeding of the five thousand and of his subsequent sending of his disciples on a field trip while he went up on a mountainside to pray, offered us this thought: "Prayer is as necessary after a triumph as it is before a difficulty." It led me to thinking.

In the twilight of my life, as I reflect on all that has gone on during the course of my living, and as I think of each day with its stress-free blessings, I think of how fortunate I have been. I have had my health; a wonderful family; a friend or two who have given sparkle to my days; a life on a job that was productive and, though sometimes difficult, was an enjoyable and satisfying one—a life that was filled with more high points than low ones. And now, in the twilight, a life that is filled with even more blessings. Each day, as I close my eyes, I can only think of how wonderful it has been. I can spend a few minutes after my head hits the pillow, reflecting on the course of the day, and go to sleep with a smile on my face.

I was taught—somewhere, sometime—that before one goes to sleep, I ought to relive the events of the day now past to see if there was anyone whom I offended and whom I should contact the next day to ask for forgiveness. Sadly, as I write these words, I think of several individuals whose friendship I lost because I did not do that. Good friends who became anything but friends because of one incident or another. Oh, if I could only go back and talk to them. Alas, however, they are gone; or in the language of our day, "passed on!" We had such good times together, but I lost those moments because of some dumb exchange of words or because of a misunderstanding; or because in some instances, I did something to them, and they chose to turn their face in another direction and I didn't do anything about it.

I remember reading of Catherine Marshall—the wife of the famed preacher Peter Marshall—who, on what she supposed was her deathbed (she got better and outlived her husband), wrote letters to a number of people whom she had offended. She wanted their forgiveness before she died. It did not say, once she recovered, if she sent the letters and what the response from them might have been.

The point is, in these latter days, there is a need to rethink the events of each day to make sure that we take advantage of the time we have left to restore any relationships that we have destroyed, for one reason or another, or allowed to be destroyed.

Oh, what a blessing my life is; and no matter what the future may be, I can only be thankful for all that I have had and all that I have… How about you?

Twenty-Three

We Need to Know The Importance of Maintaining Our Relationships!

One special thought has dawned upon me in the course of the last week or so. It has to do with the incidents in my life which affected my relationship with others and the subsequent separation from some of them because of something I said or did or something they said or did: usually it was the former. At that particular moment in time, we went our own separate ways, and now, as I write, I realize that I allowed those situations to break off good friendships and separate me from others whom I liked and admired. Sadly, in the case of two men I am thinking about, it was a "forever separation," since they have long since passed away.

In the final chapter of his book, *Too Soon Old, Too Late Smart*, Gordon Livingston writes, "Certainly, it is true that understanding who we are depends on paying attention to the history of our lives." Sometimes, between ignoring the past and wallowing in it, there is a place where we can learn from what has happened to us, including the inevitable mistakes we have made; and we can integrate this knowledge into our plans for the future. Inevitably, and we must understand this, no matter what it costs, this process will sometimes require some exercises of forgiveness. We might have to straighten up our backs, hitch up our belts, and say to someone face-to-face, "I'm sorry!" In the situations mentioned above, I did not do that, and I will be forever sorry!

It has become a custom in our family—and not a good one, I might add—to send Christmas cards each year to those from whom we heard the previous year and, usually, only to them. In other words, we give our friends two chances: respond to our card, or stop getting one. Sometimes, I am sure, addresses are lost. However, even if we lose their address, they probably didn't lose ours; so we ought to get a card from them. Otherwise, *snip*!

Maybe a card sent the next year to those we did not hear from the preceding Christmas ought to bear a note: "We didn't hear from you last year. Is something wrong?" Possibly a phone call needs to be made to solidify a relationship or renew a friendship. We have not done that, and now I am the one who worries about it. When I read those words of Livingston's quoted above, I wrote these words on the top of the page. "Stop! Reflect! Think! Act!" The next time I have my kids together, that is one bit of wisdom I want to share with them. They are still early enough in their lives that they can recapture relationships that, perhaps, have been lost. Probably not significant ones, but ones that have played a particular role in the history of their lives.

For me, most situations have become final, as mentioned above, because the people involved have passed on. However, there are some that I can still contact, and there are parts of my life's history that I can write "completed" and "satisfied" over. Why is it that we are *Too Soon Old, Too Late Smart*?

Twenty-Four

We Need to Decide What We Want to Do with the Rest of Our Lives?

I was reading someone's commentary on the life of Thomas Merton. In it, they speak of many of the unsaintly things that inflicted themselves on this holy man's life. He then makes this assessment: "The greatest gift of Merton's private journals (not published at his request until twenty-five years after his death) is to show us that even our gurus go through darkness in seeking the light, and in our spiritual failures, we are not alone."

There is a certain redemptive quality in this statement. How many things have we done in our lives of which we are not very proud? On the other hand, how many times have those very same "dark acts" later become a special blessing? How many times, after we have done things that we would really like to forget and hope never see the light of day—how many times have those very same acts become special in the days, weeks, months, and years that have followed? Hidden events have given us something that we would not have achieved or received anywhere else. Oh, we could fantasize about them, but to experience them in the flesh—wow!

Without our imagination, how poor our lives would be! How many things have we achieved in our dreams that have evaded us in real life? And the reason that they have not become real, I wonder; is it because we are too humble and afraid to be more aggressive and bring attention to ourselves, or is it because we have distanced ourselves from those things that might allow them to become a reality? And another thought: if we had achieved what we have dreamed about, how many important things would we have missed because they would have been overlooked or not experienced in our journey toward whatever we thought was worth dreaming about and working for?

Now in the latter years of life, our dreams have diminished in size because we have only the present to look forward to. Now for the most part, we focus our attention not on what we might attain, but on what we have attained! In the second half of life, too many of us have come to believe that a bird in hand *is* worth two in the bush! It is because of this conservative way of thinking that we are missing some of the excitement that might be ours if we were willing to reach out to those things that are just beyond our grasp. We are afraid to reach, for fear we will fall or maybe fail! So what if we fall once in a while? So what if we fail once in a while?

We have the opportunity to spend each minute of each hour one at a time, investing them in a happy life. We don't have the luxury of thinking about next week or next month or next year thinking only about what we *will* do! Now we can only think of what we *can* do! But then, is there not a certain freedom in that?

It goes back to the subject of discipline; something we have thought about in the past. I have an hour left, but what will I do with it? I have a day left, but what will I do with it? I have a week left, but what will I do with it? I have a year left, but what will I do with it? I have the rest of my life left, but what should I do with it? That, my friend, is the big question. What should I do with the rest of my life? Well, sit down and plan it out, and then do it. Don't leave anything more to chance because suddenly this life will end, and who will be the lesser for it? Me? You? The worlds in which we live? Give it some thought. The question is worth answering...

Twenty-Five

We Need to Believe That the Best Years of Our Life Are in Front of Us!

Finishing Well is a writing composed by Bob Buford that speaks of life in three parts: "life I," "halftime," and "life II." A description of what he means by those terms is included in the writing mentioned above. It is a book written to those who have entered the second phase of their lives, following their work lives or close to and after "halftime," a period of time when they begin to prepare for the finish line. In his words of introduction, he writes: "In the past, people thought you retired and then you died. We have choices today we've never had before. In many ways, we can make the best of our life the rest of our life."

Further, he says, "Halftime used to be the beginning of the end. Now it is the beginning of a whole new beginning." When asked at the age of seventy-eight, "Are you thinking about retiring?," the famed salesman Zig Ziglar responded, "No! I am refiring!"

Buford then presents this question, "Do you see your best years ahead of you or behind you? If people see their best years behind them, then they're probably not going to finish well because you can't finish well when you're looking backward." Ken Blanchard suggests that during the period following "halftime," we need to get under God's agenda and out from under our own. "Success," he writes, "is all about getting significance. Significance is about giving back. Ultimately, you're surrendering to God's plan for your life."

And that is all well and good, but this presupposed that during "life I," you were primarily getting and enjoying life with all its luxuries, physically and monetarily speaking, centering upon ourselves and not upon others. So in "life II," we move our focus from ourselves and put it on the people who are about us. However, what if you spent "life I" focusing on others; on giving yourself to others?

The presumption is that, that is to be the focus of "life II" as well. Frankly, however, one can get tired of spending one's life on others; that is, until you encounter a Mother Teresa, whom I have just encountered as I write this paragraph. Others were always the focus of her life, which means—if her model is valid at all—that for some of us, "life II" is to be just an extension of "life I." Now I have no problem with that thought except that a little bit of self-pity sometimes creeps in from time to time, and I have to deal with it. Frankly, pity parties are hard to avoid.

Maybe "halftime" is when you count the blessings you enjoyed during "life I" and, cognizant of them, find yourself able to launch out into "life II," looking for new worlds to conquer and new lives to mentor as you share yourself with the world around you...

So I have to stand back, count my blessings, and look forward to some new directions that will be put in my path by the Creator, God. I read! I listen! I look! I wait! And all the time, I am wondering, What does life—what does God have in store for me today or tomorrow or...?

Twenty-Six

We Can All Enter the Season of Beginning Again!

In the writing, *Spring: A Spiritual Biography of The Season*, the writers offer this thought in the preface:

> "Spring is the season that simultaneously calls us to celebration and to a sober sense of gratitude for the time that we have been given. The grace of renewal should lead to gratitude for the newness, and it should lead us to an acute awareness of our need for renewal!"

Then several pages later, in the introduction, they write, "Spring begins not with a kettledrum but with the notes of the piccolo," and "The stirrings of spring prompt expectations and hopes but also a measure of humility, because who can know what lies in front of us?"

Spring, annually, becomes a season of beginning again. It must, however, be a very personal thing. We can't steal somebody else's season. We must, rather, make it our own. I saw someone, with scissors in hand, stealing—yes, stealing—some daffodils from a public landscaped approach to our road this afternoon. With a nonchalance born, I would suspect, out of ignorance or lack of any sense of ethic, the individual stopped their car, opened the door, and deftly cut some flowers that belonged to all the rest of us. They then drove their car away, undoubtedly very proud of themselves for stealing something from someone else. Another mark of our time?

Be that as it may, it reminded me that we cannot steal someone else's spring, no matter how nonchalant we may appear to be. We have to make our own spring. We must listen for the music of the piccolo and then add in our own notes of joy and help, and help to produce a time of renewal for ourselves and, likely, for those around us.

What does it take to bring springtime into our lives? A time of reflection, blotting out the winters of our discontent and trouble? A time for a renewed vision when we see not the dead leaves of the autumn now past and the winter but the new buds as they appear on tree and ground. Within every bud lies the opportunity of a new life, a new adventure, a new beginning. Within each one of them lies the opportunity to move out in another direction, having left the crossroads to walk one way or another, while our old life stops or walks forward in a new direction.

As the spring dawns and the season of Lent travels fast to its conclusion, we all have the chance to look back on what we have done and what we have not done, throw the dirt of time on it, and then dig a new hole into which we can place the fresh seed of a new beginning.

There is really something wonderful to be found in planting a new seed or plant and watching it play its role on the landscape of our lives. I hear the sound of the piccolo, and hey, isn't that the sound of some new expectation, desire, or dream reaching itself out of the new fresh and warm soil of another season?

Twenty-Seven

We Need to Deal with the Problem of Our Procrastination!

Speaking of the problem or danger of being a procrastinator, a writer offers up this defense or cure: "One of the best escapes from the prison of procrastination is to take even the smallest step toward your goal." I have been stricken with the disease or problem of procrastination, whatever you might call it, at periodic times in my life, so I found the words being addressed to me.

It is so easy to sit down in the morning or evening and make plans for the day ahead—great plans, idealistic plans—and then not carry them out. "I will begin tomorrow morning!" However, when tomorrow comes, I don't follow through on the plans that I have made. Rather, I say, "I think I will begin tomorrow morning!" The problem has been "tomorrow never seems to come," and life goes on, on its merry way, with no change or development.

I came across this short poem entitled, "9:00–9:15 AM"

> "I've dusted my desk and I've wound up my watch,
> I've tightened (then loosened) my belt by a notch.
> I've polished my glasses, removed a small speck,
> I've looked at my check stubs to check on a check.
> I've searched for my tweezers, and pulled out a hair,

I've opened a window to let in some air.
I've straightened a picture, I've swatted a fly,
I've shifted the tie clip that clips on my tie.
I've sharpened each pencil till sharp as a dirk,
I've run out of reasons for not starting work."

Procrastination is the enemy of discipline. Discipline is something that people, like myself, do not seem to be able to handle or practice or... We have talked a number of times about to-do lists. Having things written down and doing what is written down in the order of its appearance. Maybe there is a need to start at the beginning.

My name is _____, and I am a procrastinator!

I have never been much of a list maker. Maybe I need to become one. I think it is probably worth a try since all I have been writing about is discipline, and even when I practice a daily regimen, there is much that remains to be done; and there are items, daily items, that never seem to get done. The problem is, at this time in my life, if they are not being done, very likely, they will not get done.

Now the world will never miss my doing those things, but my life will. I need the prideful sense of accomplishment that comes from crossing things off my list: of dotting the "i's" and crossing the "t's!" I know that some of those same things will appear in my life again, and I will have to put them on a new list; but that is okay. At least I will deal with them now. Let tomorrow take care of its own. So here's to making a list, here's to checking it twice, and here's to beginning to do those things that are on that list!

My name is _____, and I am going to stop being a procrastinator; and if a list is how I am going to accomplish my goal, I am going to start making a list. Let's see what happens!

Twenty-Eight

It Is Important That We Be Prepared!

The advertisement placed by a nationally known investment company (Edward Jones) showed a man caught in the rapids of a river, sitting on a small plastic pool cushion, with a drink on a plastic table beside him. He had a bewildered look on his face because he didn't know how he got there. The ad read: "Not being prepared for retirement doesn't make much sense either." Down the page was this cover statement: "One minute you've got plenty of time to prepare for retirement. The next minute, you're struggling to keep your head above water."

Another company is offering a "dream book" to would-be investors. It, too, or so the television commercial declares, will "assist you in planning your tomorrows." Both advertisements want to speak to us about "being financially ready for our retirement," for that period in our life when we will have the opportunity to enjoy the things that we have not had the chance to do because of the confines of our labor and our growing family.

Maybe! I say that because I am not sure that a lot of people are looking forward today to their retirement. Many, maybe most people, fret a bit about the extent of their financial resources as they look ahead to those days of leisure. For them, the important question is, "Will I have enough money to cover my needs in those many extra years that I hope lie ahead of me?"

Then I remembered a conversation I had with an acquaintance on the golf course many years ago. He had just sold his company to a Fortune 100 Corporation, had built a second home in Arizona, and was anticipating the winter months in that place. His comment stopped me: "You know you can only play so much golf." It dawned on me then, and I think about it now, but there is more to retirement than financial security. I might add that the man to whom I was talking died prematurely, maybe from a lack of purpose in his life.

In other words, retirement is not an age thing; it is a state-of-mind thing. All the money in the world cannot fill your days with enjoyment and satisfaction. How many men and women do I know—did I know—who retired and died? Their lives hit a wall of inactivity that they could not handle. Aggressive, busy, productive—and then? I had another friend, an executive in a large oil company. On the first day of his retirement, his wife called him into the kitchen and said, "Paul! You retired! I didn't. Every morning, around ten, I sit down at the kitchen table with a cup of coffee and the morning paper, and I don't want to see your face!" It was not a mad remark. It was a statement of concern. In other words, "Paul, get a life. Get a new life!" He did, at the time, but a number of years later, he committed suicide.

There is more to retirement than financial security. The fact of the matter is, when you hit the magic age, no matter what it may be, you had better have made some plans to make your future days more enjoyable and satisfactory. You may be at that point today; maybe the day is coming tomorrow? The point is, you have got some planning to do. "Not being prepared for retirement doesn't make much sense!" Remember, today is the first day of the rest of your life! Hopefully, it will be a long one filled with joy and satisfaction along with financial security. "Get a life! A new life!"

Twenty-Nine

You Need to Grow the Leader That Is within You!

No one of us knows what we are capable of doing until we are challenged to marshal our strengths and bring them forward. Activist and author Rita Mae Brown says it like this: "People are like tea bags. You never know how strong they'll be until you put them into hot water."

Writing in their book, *A Leader's Legacy*, authors James Kouzes and Barry Posner remind us that "all leaders are born," following up with these words: "We've never met a leader who wasn't (born)." We're all born. So? It's what you do with what you have before you die that's important. Furthermore, they write, "Somewhere, sometime, the leader within each of us will get the call to step forward. By believing in ourselves and by developing our capacity to lead, we'll be prepared when that call comes. And each time we accept a call, we are saying yes to one more opportunity that will help us to leave a lasting legacy in the worlds where we live and work and play."

No one of us knows how many calls we will receive to exercise our gifts in our service of self and sour fellow human beings. In this day and age with careers starting and stopping, with opportunities opening up almost daily, each one of us can decide the impact we will have on the worlds around us. We can become couch potatoes, or we can jump into some boiling water and become what we were intended to become.

When I was in graduate school in Pittsburgh, there was a traffic cop who was made famous by a television station that chronicled his actions during the evening rush hour. He was a master at directing traffic at a busy downtown intersection. He made a lot of his job, and no one could tell how much he enjoyed it. They knew he did; they just did not know how much he loved it.

Who knows what possibilities lie within our being? Often we find ourselves confined by our jobs and by the limited opportunities that are available to us during our working years. It is only later, when we have been freed of our obligations and of the environment in which we originally placed ourselves, that we find the chance to unfurl our real selves and benefit the worlds in which we live.

I encountered a greeter at a local Walmart Store who put a smile on my face when I went shopping one day. Now, I am not a "happy shopper;" I usually do it rather reluctantly, but on that particular day, I did my required duty with a smile in my heart. My Walmart hostess brightened up my day, and all she said was, "Good afternoon!" I don't know anything about her background or about what she did before she assumed her place before that entry door. However, she filled a special niche in a lot of lives. She did her job with gusto, and I remember her to this day...

What are the hidden gifts that have been placed within us? Kouzes and Posner write, "In more than twenty years of research, we've been fortunate to have heard and read the stories of thousands of ordinary people who've led others to get extraordinary things done. Ordinary people whose names are not known and whose stories are not told in the daily news. There are millions more! It's not the absence of leadership potential that inhibits the development of more leaders. It's the persistence of the myth that leadership can't be learned. The haunting myth is a far more powerful deterrent to leadership development than is the nature of the person or the basics of the leadership process."

Who knows what potential lies with me or you? We just have to find an environment that will enable us to let it out. It takes a lot of time and a bit of reflection and thought, but it is there to be used again and again in one way or another. Where and how will you leave your mark on the world?

THIRTY

It Is Important That We Have Some Priorities in Our Lives!

Spring is in the air, though winter is endeavoring to fight one more battle to show its supremacy over nature. And what a tough season it was. Not a whole lot of snow, but a great deal of damage, evident everywhere. Mostly leaf damage caused by leaves that were not picked up and by the moisture that made them a death blanket over grass and plant of every kind. It is that time of year we call "cleanup time!" It is the time of year that I like the least. The desolation of the winter months, the blue days of January and February; suddenly they are gone, and the springtime of April and May are, all at once, upon us.

The problem with such a situation and the "retired person" is that my bones and body are no longer adequate to the tasks in front of me. The mind is willing, but the body is weak! Bending and picking up things is not really an option. Whereas in the old days, when I was younger, I could work endlessly at such tasks as weeding, raking, planting, and pruning; now they are an undertaking that is almost overwhelming. Like life, one needs others to help in the accomplishment of the many tasks presented during "the cleanup season!" Yes, I can do one little job a day, but that is so frustrating to someone who wants things done *yesterday*! This is one of the reasons that I hated to paint and paper. Too much time had to be wasted in doing the preparatory tasks. By the time I was ready to paper or paint or both,

I didn't want to do it anymore. The body was willing, but the mind had moved on to other interests.

But be that as it may, nature beckons. So as with every aspect of life, one has to plan. What are my plans for each area in my domain, and how will I accomplish the necessary tasks to satisfy my expectations? I must admit that during the working days of my life, I did too often a minimum amount of work. I had so many dreams, but I did not do all the things that needed to be done to accomplish them. Now, today, I have the time, but I no longer have the required energy to do all that I want to do. As I write, I am thinking about how I will piece together all of my resources to accomplish my plans.

It is, as I suggested, like the second half of life: the mind is willing, but body and resources are somewhat limited. So as with life, there is the need to take nature on one step at a time. First the division of my labors into digestible units. Plan and schedule! Then secondly, *doing the discipline necessary to accomplish them.* Time is not the issue. I have the time. The problem is setting my priorities.

Yes, it will take some time—some valuable time—and I know that I do not have a lot of it. It will require dealing with my impatience; with my desire to get things done today and not tomorrow. We might call it "pausing for effect!" We never have time to waste, but we waste a lot of time because too often we do not wisely plan how to use our minutes, hours, days and weeks. Wasted time! We all know what that is about! The later years demand that we stand back from our lives and plan every minute of them. There is great satisfaction in accomplishing our intended tasks. However, sometimes we are so intent on the ends that we don't spend our attention on the means to attain that end.

I am going somewhere. I am not sure when I will arrive at my destination, maybe never, but I look forward to the adventure. Now *time-out*: I am going to do some planning! World! Watch out! I am coming!

THIRTY-ONE

We Have to Determine for Ourselves the Things That Matter!

In one of his more recent writings entitled, *Eat This Book*, Eugene Peterson offers up this thought: "If we try to understand and form ourselves by ourselves, we leave out most of ourselves." His thesis is, of course, from a Christian point of view: that we need to find and develop a personal relationship with Jesus Christ because as we open ourselves up to him, God will show us who we are, why we are, and what we should be becoming. It is imperative, from Peterson's point of view, that we are not to conform the will and way of God to ourselves, but quite the reverse: we are to conform ourselves to the will and way of God. Ours is a life of conformance, and the meaning of the question, "What would Jesus do?" is one for each one of us to understand and answer for ourselves.

In the same vein, Bob Buford, in his work, *Finishing Well*, writes, "What keeps most of us from focusing on the things that matter is all the things that don't matter, but add cost, particularly the cost of our most precious asset, *our time*." In reference to another person's philosophy, he recalls, "He's decided on what he's not going to do in order to focus on those things that he feels called to do."

We're still on the same road we were weeks ago in our retirement life. That is, assuming we know who we are, we must keep asking ourselves the question: "What do I feel called to do?" I am probably one of those few persons in the world who, at a late age with most of my life behind me and an uncertain time ahead, continues to ask the question, "What do I feel called to do?"

I continue to be bound by the disciplines of a former life and time, and I cannot get out from under them. I wonder, sometimes, if much of what I do really matters, or if I am just doing life in the wrong way because I do not know how to do it any other way?

It is far beyond halftime, to paraphrase Buford, so I guess I need to call a time-out, and maybe another one, to allow me the opportunity to have the time necessary to again think about developing a game plan that will point me in the right direction. What are the things that matter at this juncture in my life? What am I doing that is consuming that precious commodity called "my time"? Oh, how I wish I knew…

A walk in the woods? A retreat that would enable me to really think through where I am and what I want to do? The ability to cast off from the shore of my past and present disciplines to find a new way, a new adventure, a satisfactory enterprise?

It is a daily task, this process of determining where I am and where I want to go. Every hour is important; every day a very special opportunity to continue on my present journey or deviate and travel in another direction. The need—at least, as far as I am concerned—is to utilize every minute in the time that I have left in life to satisfy my best intentions and create a sense of accomplishment within myself.

Thirty-Two

There Is a Need to Satisfy Our Passions!

I came across this phrase in my reading the other day: "The point of passion is mainly to follow: to let yourself love what you love, or respect your hunger and obey your thirst." It got me to thinking about my past, my present, and my future, however long it will be. When I was growing up, my father, who was an educator, never found time, it seemed, to read. Oh, I am sure that he did it professionally in small doses during the day in his office, but our house didn't have many books; they just weren't there, and if they were there, they were not visible. We used the library, or at least I did, a lot; but our house didn't even have a bookshelf. Then when he retired, I found that even though I tried to tempt him into doing some reading, it didn't work. It truly made me sad. One book I bought him, later in life, I know was never opened even though he tried to tell me of his interest in it. It is now on *my* bookshelf—still unread, I might add.

I have always loved books. I love to rummage through the bookstores available to me. I buy too many books. The shelves behind the chair in which I am sitting are bulging with many books that I have had ever since I retired eight years ago. They were bought to be read and researched, to provide me with some professional advice. I had determined, when I bought them, that I would be able to use them to give substance and zest to the institution which I served. Now there are additional piles of books purchased in recent weeks and months, waiting to be picked up and read on the floor in front of the bookshelves. I must admit that I am a "bookaholic!" I love to read! For what purpose, I don't know. I guess the fact of the matter is, I just love to buy books to possess them—to have them available when I want to read them.

And then I read the above-quoted phrase. "The point of passion is mainly to follow: to let yourself love what you love, or respect your hunger and obey your thirst." Then I came upon a chapter in another book on my reading pile. Entitled *Live What You Love*, written by Bob and Melinda Blanchard, it has a chapter entitled, "The Big 4." In it, these words:

> "Beginnings are exciting. We dream of what will spring from our imaginations, off the stove, into the marketplace, and into our lives. We can almost taste its sweet success—whether it is a new recipe, a new building, a new business, or a new life. Along with the joy, excitement and anticipation comes the challenge. How do we do this? How do we make *this* dream a reality? How do we take everything we've learned and use it to our advantage?"

The authors point out that they have discovered four checkpoints in life that help them connect their dreams with reality. They are passion, people, environment and money; and "like the pistons in your car engine, they should all be in proper working order and running smoothly." Now they write that they try not to put more emphasis on any one of the Big 4 because "they are all important." I will!

They ask, "Do we believe in what we are doing? Are we passionate about it? Are we moving toward a life we love? You need to be honest with yourself, your expectations, and your experiences if you want to live what you love."

How important is passion? Ultimately, I think that is what life is finally all about. Passion is important! The lesson I received—or am teaching, if you will—from my reading is, I don't have to have a reason for reading. There does not have to be a purpose for it. I can just read and read and read because it makes me happy and satisfies my needs; and when my life is over, there will still be books on the floor, waiting for a reader. There does not have to be a reason to read or to do anything that really interests us, an end purpose in sight. I just need to have the passion to obey my thirst. My only requirement to be satisfied is to sit down and read and love every minute of it.

And what is your passion at this point in your life? Are you geared to satisfy it?

Thirty-Three

We Need to Think About Tomorrow!

I've heard it read at one funeral or another, these words from the pen of Henry Wadsworth Longfellow:

> As a fond mother, when the day is o'er,
> leads by the hand her little child to bed,
> half willing, half reluctant to be led,
> and leave his broken playthings on the floor,
> still gazing at them through the open door,
> nor wholly reassured and comforted
> by promises of others in their stead
> which, though more splendid, may not please
>   him more;
> So nature deals with us, and takes away
> our playthings one by one, and by the hand
> leads us to reset so gently, that we go
> scarce knowing if we wish to go or stay,
> being too full of sleep to understand
> how far the unknown transcends that what we
>   know."

Yes, we are all in the process of "going." The journey begins on the day that we were born and will progress until the day nature takes it all away from us. Someone has suggested, I know not who or when, that we cannot really be in control of our lives until we can visualize life without our being here.

A recent Daytona 500 race was won by a hundredth of a second or two. The winner of the event was asked if he had taken his foot off his accelerator as he approached the finish line. His response was, in effect, "No, we were going full bore until the end. My foot was to the floor!"

I would suggest that we need to do two things as we enter the third stage of our living. First we must come to grips with the realization that there is an end time to this thing we call life and that we need to live all of our lives. In other words, since the end has been in sight for all these years we have been living, let's put our pedal to the floor and make sure we live our lives out right to the end.

Nature *does* take away our playthings one by one. We don't move as fast as we did at one time. We have aches and pains that we could not have imagined, even a year or so ago. We don't run up and down the stairs as quickly as before, but be that as it may, to use the words of a philosopher, "we are not homesick" because there is still too much living for us to do before we lay down for the final time.

We don't have to think about our limitations except to make allowances for them in the way we live. Rather, we have to think about the possibilities that are still within us and endeavor to realize them in the days, weeks, months, and years ahead of us.

So as I have, push that accelerator pedal to the floor and make plans to cross the finish line at full speed.

Thirty-Four

We Must Endure the Punishment of Impatience!

Nikos Kazantzakis is best known to the world as the author of *Zorba the Greek*. In his autobiography, which he entitled, *Report to Greco*, he tells of an encounter he had one day along life's road. He came upon a cocoon cradled in the bark of an olive tree just as the butterfly was making a hole and attempting to emerge. Impatient for results, he bent over it and warmed it under his breath, planning, he anticipated, to speed up the process. The butterfly, however, emerged prematurely; its wings hopelessly crumpled and stuck to its own body. It needed the patient warmth of the sun's rays and not the impertinent breath of a man to transform it. Moments later, after a desperate struggle, the butterfly died in the palm of his hand.

"That little body," he wrote later, "is the greatest weight I have on my conscience."

Impatience! It is the scourge of many an older person, and I am one of them. Perhaps it is because life has an imminent end, and as the years pass, that particular time looms on the horizon. As a result, we don't have time to wait; we want to see results *now*!

It is springtime. It is that time of the year when nature needs some assistance in preparing for the splendor of summer. Leaves need to be raked. Bushes need to be trimmed! Grass needs to be cut, and the damage of winter, in general, healed. It is something that requires time to plan and accomplish. It demands patience! One needs to make plans for the summer! Plant flowers and grass seeds. Make changes in the decor of the landscape. Have the chance to create, and then step back and enjoy one's work. It needs patience.

I have always been impatient, perhaps because a heavy work schedule interfered in the aforementioned processes. But now—even though the years are slowly passing—too fast in our retirement years, we have the chance to slow down the process and enjoy it every step of the way. Now we can watch the bushes "green-up" bud and flower. Now we can plan and then remake the plan.

And so with life. Now no one seems to be able to wait even for a minute for something to happen. We need to learn to live today and not tomorrow. Forget much of the past, and live in the present. What a wonderful time of life is to be found in its later years. To plan and to reflect; to look and to do! Put out the chair! Find a good book and a place to put one's feet. Turn on the music and enjoy all that nature has to offer. Plan and accomplish! Live today and not worry about tomorrow. Something will happen in this life *or* the next. Patience is a virtue to be practiced and enjoyed!

Thirty-Five

The Importance of Yesterday's Memories!

The raspberry patch is gone! I discovered this reality while I was cutting my grass this afternoon. It has been there for as long as I have lived in the house where I live. It had been nurtured by my neighbor. It was a small patch with only a few plants, just enough to provide him and his wife with five to ten small servings during the season.

He nurtured it! He fertilized it! He relished its becoming and enjoyed the harvest. Once in a while he gave us some. But now it is gone. However, so is my neighbor! First his wife left this world of reality: several years before she died, the dreaded Alzheimer's disease taking her past and present and fiendishly emptying her memory. Then my neighbor moved into a small condominium. It was there that he died. Now the patch is gone—the new property owners having dug it up and disposed of it. Now no one will remember it except me. Then I will be gone, and the bare ground will be swallowed up by grass and weeds; and its presence there will have been extinguished forever.

The process is not unlike leaving one's job after a lifetime of labor. Suddenly a desk chair is empty, a desk is cleaned out, and everything left in it is disposed of by the new occupant of the chair. It is not long, and then no one remembers who had been seated there before. On another day, the desk will be moved or replaced with a new one, and the chair dispatched to another location.

And all that went into the process called life: it will be gone. But that is life! We live it. We cherish it! We value it far more than others, and then something new is to be seen and found and the past is forgotten.

It means that each one of us must cherish what we have, enjoy the product of our labors, taste what is good, and relish it; because in the not-too-distant future, life will change, take on a new course, and then…

It is said that beauty is in the eye of the beholder! And so is much of our lives. We value things. We work to accomplish our goals and our dreams. We enjoy our Andy Warhol moments in the sun, and we should do just that. But our lives move on, and one day, all too soon, almost everything about it will be forgotten.

My neighbor enjoyed the raspberries! I appreciated the diligence which he gave to their raising and consumption. Vicariously, I felt his joy and satisfaction; not as much as he did, I am sure, but I was a bystander and, therefore, a participant in this particular enterprise in his life.

And what about my yard and my house and the things that I hold dear? One day, whoever lives in this place will not know who was here before them. They will find separate joys and satisfaction in this house and its surrounding yard. How wonderful, because I have found such joy and satisfaction in this house and its surrounding environs. I know they will too, and there is some significant satisfaction in that as well.

Life *is* a fleeting moment in time, and I am thankful for all that is mine and all that I have found enjoyable in it. Tomorrow something new will happen. I will forget much of what has happened today. However, I have a chance to relish each accomplishment and anticipate each new day and each new project, because that is God's gift to me, just as that raspberry patch was a gift to my neighbor and me!

Thirty-Six

We All Need Encouragement, Enthusiasm, and Excitement in Our Lives!

We all need to listen to or to read of the excitement for life that is registered by one motivational speaker or writer or another in their presentations, audible or written. We need to be captured by the enthusiasm that they bring to life's table. When we were young, we were constantly encouraged to apply extra effort to excel in our studies, in our vocations, and in our extracurricular activities. How-to talks were constantly sent in our direction. Now today, some of us, as we are treading time in what Bob Buford calls the "halftime or second half of our lives," need some additional encouragement and motivation. We need to again listen and consider the possibilities being presented to us by those same speakers and writers or their twenty-first century counterparts.

One such offering is a book entitled *The Magic of Thinking Big*. The writer, David Schwartz, writes that anyone who is bored by life has probably forgotten his or her dreams. He then, in the pages that he has written, invites his readers to get back in touch with themselves. As a first step, he asks us to list all the things that we have ever wanted to accomplish. I was introduced to Mr. Schwartz's book by Coach Lou Holtz in a collection of writings found in the writing, *You've Got to Read This Book*. (See bibliography.)

Coach Holtz writes that Schwartz challenged him to write down a list of his hopes and dreams. He (Holtz) divided his list into five categories:

1. As a husband/father
2. Spiritually
3. Professionally
4. Financially
5. Simply for excitement

Holtz concludes: "From the time I made the list [and completed it], I became a participant rather than a spectator in my life. You do the same thing, and you'll find out you don't want to spend much time sleeping. You'll be afraid you might miss something."

At my stage in life, categories 3 and 4 are, for the most part, already documented and completed; though in some small way, this writing is a play on number 3. However, categories 1, 2, and 5 are still under development. Holtz said that he let his imagination run wild when it came to the fifth category. You'll have to read the book mentioned above to get a small taste of his list, but it is an exciting read.

Life, in any one of its time periods, can be filled with excitement, success, and fulfillment. There is so much ahead of us. It should never have to be boring. I know it isn't for me. Maybe there is danger, however, in letting your wife and kids read the items you have placed under the first category?

Thirty-Seven

We Need to Take the Time to Relax and Regroup!

As I was reading today, the thought came to me that in the course of my working lifetime, usually I took one day off each week. It was normally Friday, and I expended it either playing golf or working at home. Today, as I read a chapter in Greg Levoy's book, *Callings*, I was brought up short by some words he was destined to put in front of me.

Levoy speaks of finding a time in his life following the completion of a book, when he reached "burnout!" He hit a wall and found himself utterly bankrupt of energy, finding himself almost buckling at the knees. He writes that he determined to take a period of time off. In his case, it was to be a four-month period when he would live off his savings, etc.

He writes: "For my entire leave of absence,"—I like that phrase—"I experienced a bewildering freedom, marked by a maddening restlessness that, despite my best intentions, routinely propelled me, as if I were in a trance, back into my office. There I would sit, sometimes for hours, twisting back and forth in my chair and pulling up my lower lip, listening to the blathering traffic of many noises in my head, my legs vibrating like tuning forks under the desk."

Then he wrote the words that gripped my attention: "This is what it must be like when men retire." It is something that I have mentioned before in these writings. His rational for the above-quoted paragraph: "Value adheres to what we produce, so we're constantly doing. When we're busy doing, we don't have time to be busy feeling." The point that he wished to make, I assume, was, "When we are retired, we have time for feeling!"

Then he speaks to the reward of his leave of absence. "Sitting quietly, hushing for even a few minutes a day, gives us a place in which to catch our breath and a chance for our callings and intuitions to catch up with us. Just as the ear needs rest when we are listening to music, or the eye and the mind need the respite of occasional paragraph breaks when reading a book, we all need a place where we can linger and reflect in the onrushing of our story or song, an eddy into which we can turn our canoe from the current."

Well, springtime has arrived in my life in the midst of my encountering retirement, and with it, the outside beckons. Work in the yard. Weeding and recovering the landscape from the winter. Planting, sitting out on the deck with a good book, playing golf—whatever! It is time to reassess my schedule and embark on some new activities.

I guess I should have been doing this my whole lifetime through, but I was always too involved to take the time to linger and think about my future. Now in the leisure of retirement and all its vacant but fertile days, I can do just that, and I began doing it today! Hurray! I have finally grown up to what life ought to be about. It is a time of reflection, of coming to terms with my feelings, of thinking about tomorrow in the midst of my todays.

Life is for living, and living demands that we recognize who we are and what we ought to be about. Then and only then do we have the opportunity to realize all the possibilities that life can present to us, and the realization that if we plan wisely and life treats us well, we will have the chance to do most of them!

Thirty-Eight

It Is Always Time to Begin Again!

A while ago, after I retired for the third time, I gave away all the accumulated books in my library assembled over a professional lifetime: forty-plus years; well-over four thousand books. I thought a younger man would benefit from my years of accumulation and from my labors. Included in the gift was a filing system that documented the reading I had done as well as file drawers full of materials that I had gathered over time, pertinent to particular subjects and concerns. I also gave to that recipient some newly purchased office furniture I had bought to furnish my retirement office in an uptown location. That furniture included the proverbial desk, a credenza, several filing cabinets, and bookshelves sufficient to house all the books.

In the years that have followed, the young man to whom I gave what I considered a treasure trove of resources and information of significant worth has often called to tell me how much he appreciated the furniture. However, never once, in all our conversations, has he ever referred to the books, etc. Now they were the primary purpose of my gift to him. But he has never mentioned them; never once.

I had placed at his disposal material that had been a blessing to me and, I am sure, to others, over forty and more years of labor. I sometimes wonder if others would have received what was given in much the same way? Some material objects, some office furniture, and nothing more? I must admit that often I have wanted to ask him what he did with the books, files, and the other cerebral materials. However, I have never had the courage or desire to do that, fearing, I suspect, that they have been given away or discarded.

I have always loved to find myself in the midst of the minds of other men and women to hear them think and write. I am just reading a book on the life of the Roman Catholic priest, Henri Nouwen. His was a life of contemplation and sharing. I will never be in his league—not even in the minor leagues, far below him—but I have been blessed by his thoughts. Biography and autobiography are a resource of unbelievable depth and mental fulfillment.

I have often wondered if I just like to accumulate books, read or unread.? However, as I read Nouwen, I sadly, again, become aware of my grief. A whole library forgotten, lost in the midst of some accumulated but not too expensive office furniture. How could someone miss all that knowledge and not want to jump in and begin to read, let alone use it?

Now again, I find myself beginning, again, to buy books. My study is filling up with new books. Frankly, now there is now no ultimate purpose in reading them other than to plumb the depths of one mind or another and enjoy the fruits of other thinkers. But I must admit, I wonder, where will these books go after I am gone? Who will plunder or use them? I hope their recipient will do better.

Thirty-Nine

We Need to Listen and Hear Words of Wisdom from the Past!

The other day, I chanced upon a small book entitled, *The Fred Factor*, written by Mark Sanborn. It contains a whole lot of interesting stuff! For example, these words attributed to basketball coach John Wooden's father, Joshua. The elder Wooden is quoted as saying, "Make each day your masterpiece!" Another chapter is prefaced by these words of Abraham Lincoln. "Whatever you are, be a good one."

Sanborn writes, "Nobody can prevent you from choosing to be exceptional." He then quotes these words of Martin Luther King Jr.: "If a man is called to be a street sweeper, he should sweep streets even as Michelangelo painted or Beethoven composed music or Shakespeare wrote poetry. He should sweep streets so well that all of the hosts of heaven and earth will pause to say, 'Here lived a great street sweeper who did his job well.'" He then closes the chapter by concluding, "I believe that no matter what job you hold, what industry you work in, or where you live, every morning you wake up with a clean slate. You can make your business, as well as your life, anything you choose it to be." That's what is called "The Fred Factor." The theory holds true for every day and every experience in your life.

"You can make your life anything that you choose it to be." Again, we are talking about dreams. We ought never to lose them. We ought always to be in search of the satisfaction of old dreams and the creation of new ones. My thesis is: that is what retirement is all about! Satisfying old dreams and creating new ones!

And as you dream your dreams and ponder their fulfillment and satisfaction, "whatever you are, be a good one." So how do I positively satisfy my accumulated dreams? There are so many that I have put in escrow, waiting for the chance when I would have the time to do them and seek to maintain the exuberance and enthusiasm that would allow me to see them through to their fulfillment.

Life is all about dreams! I know it! You know it! The danger is that we will sacrifice them at the altar of frustration and indifference and never see them fulfilled, let alone tried! Sanborn presents these words from the mind of Fred Smith: "Most people have a passion for significance. The fact of the matter is, we all have a passion for significance; the problem is, many of us don't have an enduring passion, so we stop and get off from our 'dream express' somewhere short of the goal."

Please don't ever fall victim to a pessimistic thought that will talk you out of any one of your dreams! As long as you have breath—as long as you have a mind that thinks and a body that, in one way or another, works—your dreams are within your grasp. Do them!

FORTY

We Need to Learn How to Live Life Number 2! It Is a Little Different Than Life Number 1

A long time ago, I don't remember when or why, a friend gave me a reflective book by a woman by the name of Doris Grumbach. In the preface to her writing, she offered this thought: "For some years, I have looked at guidebooks, how-to books, personal accounts, advice to the prayer life—all offering helpful hints on attempting the same expedition. They are well-intentioned, I am sure. But they violate the one rule of which I am certain: no one can act as a guide for anyone else. No way is better or best. All travelers must pack their own baggage; start out alone; travel single file; endure all the disappointments, despairs, and darknesses by themselves; and be resigned to making very slow progress. Still, as Montaigne said, 'It is not the arrival but the journey that matters.'"

Such a quest is evidenced by the writings included in this collection. The journey from one's day of retirement until the end of one's time is a very personal one. I have read and continued to read the autobiographical and biographical statements of others. How-to books—you name them, I have read them and continued to read them; though I sometimes wonder why. I guess it is because they reside on my bookshelves, and I would like to read through them all and be done with them before I close my eyes for the last time.

On the special day mentioned earlier, I began a new journey. Bob Buford calls it "life number 2." As Grumbach suggests, "There are up days and there are down days," containing both up and down moments. As I think back over the last several months, I am not sure that I have made any progress in my quest to find a new way of living or a new discipline to help me spend my days profitably, and I am finding the days can be frustratingly slow! However, I keep on trying!

So the words of Montaigne, simple but true, "It is not the arrival, but the journey that matters," intrigued me. As a result, I continue with my quest for satisfaction, internal or external, visible or invisible.

I must admit that I am enjoying the journey. Now, instead of extended thought and writing, I have brief moments of conversation with the authors whom I am reading and with myself. I am not sure that I am getting anywhere, and expect that when I get somewhere, I will not even know where I am. But I will continue to read and reflect and write and hope that one day, because I am a methodical person, I will arrive at a satisfactory way to live out each day and feel satisfied at its end.

Again, I am not sure what the purpose of the remaining years of my journey will produce, but I like Montaigne's words and will to continue to walk with Grumbach through the readings in my possession. I will probably even buy some more. I suspect that there are and will be more truths for me to consider and enjoy. Slow progress with purposeful activity. Sounds like a good formula to practice and profit by.

Let the journey continue!

FORTY-ONE

We Need to Make Hope a Living Reality in Our Lives!

I have just celebrated another birthday, one that might be called a "landmark date" in the ongoing living of my life. With its going still on my mind, I came across these words in the opening chapter of a book that I just picked off my reading shelf: "Deep down, many of us long for something that is really worthwhile. We are looking for something that really matters. There seems to be something about human nature that makes it want to long for something that is life-changing. While many people are troubled by the thoughts of dying, others are disturbed by a more profound anxiety: that they might die without having really begun to live!" The writer is Alister McGrath, and the book, *The Unknown God!*

I guess you might say that he is commenting on a truth that he felt he had uncovered several pages earlier. There he had begun, "The great certainty of our time seems to be that satisfaction is nowhere to be found. We roam around, searching without finding, yearning without being satisfied." And this one too, "Maybe we will have to get used to the fact that we are always going to fail in our search for happiness."

The conclusion, reached in regard to such a truth, comes from the pen of Robert Louis Stevenson: "To travel is better than to arrive."

There is, I think, a sadness to be found in McGrath's words: "that we might die without having really begun to live." I can honestly say that such is not the case in my life. How about yours? I remember the words of a little girl who said to a friend, "I hope that you will live all your life!" Well, that is my wish for you.

I personally have enjoyed almost every one of my days. Yes, there have been setbacks, frustrations, pain, and suffering that I have encountered in my relationship with other members of my family and with people on the outside of it, but by and large, my days have been satisfying ones. Perhaps my dreams have been limited, and my goals shortsighted; but I can look back with satisfaction on so much. I have found satisfaction. I have enjoyed a great deal of happiness.

Possibly, one of the reasons for this is that I find myself counting my accomplishments each evening as I put my head on a pillow. In the morning, now I can reflect on what I want to do during the coming day; and in the evening, I can count my blessings in the light of what I have done. Yes, I do not do some of the things that I had planned to do. However, there is always tomorrow, and if tomorrow never comes, then someone else will have to do them if they really need getting done. What was it the Gospel song said, "One day at a time, Lord Jesus, one day at a time"?

So the plan has to be to live one's life one day at a time. We need to ascertain what needs to be done *today* and do it and leave, until tomorrow, tomorrow's tasks. "To travel hopefully is a better thing than to arrive!" Yes, Robert, I am traveling hopefully, and I am satisfied that my journey has been completed no matter when it ends.

Forty-Two

The Importance of Developing a Sense of Consciousness!

The great philosopher of another day, Plato, told this insightful story. Imagine a dark cave in which a group of people had lived since they were born. They know no other world. In the cave, there is a fire burning, offering them both warmth and light. As the flames rise, they cast shadows on the walls of the cave. For those living in the cave, this world of flickering shadows is all that they know. Their grasp of reality is limited to this world. If there is a world beyond the cave, it is something which they do not know and cannot imagine. Their horizons are limited and determined by the shadows and half light provided by the fire.

Now imagine that one of that group of people huddling around that fire discovers a secret way out of the cave. He slips away unnoticed by the remainder of the group. As he explores the recesses of the cave, he stumbles across a passage hidden in the living rock, unnoticed in the darkness. He begins to explore, slowly and tentatively, moving forward and upward. Finally he emerges into some glorious sunlight, entering into a world of fresh air, green trees, blue skies, and radiant brightness. The world of flickering shadows has been left behind, and a new world is discovered.

The flickering and gloomy world of the cave was real, not imaginary. Yet the reality of that world does not call into question the possibility that there might be another world, a world which is somehow hinted at or signposted by the world we know. Our desire for something that seems never to be satisfied is one of those hints. A hint that ours is not the only world, and that true fulfillment is not to be found within it; we all have felt it, have we not?

The writer who reminded me of those words had a spiritual intent in mind. He writes, "The desire that we experience in the world can thus be thought of as a real desire for something that lies beyond the world." He is probably right in his thinking.

But more to the point, at this moment in time, could Plato also be alluding to the fact that there is so much in life that we cannot comprehend it or contain it all in our mind at the same time; that ours is a developing consciousness?

The writer also conjectures: "It is like the man who broke free from the cave and discovered a brilliant and clear new world beyond. It lifts the curtain, perhaps, only briefly on something else. Yet the glimpse, however brief, is enough to make us want more and wonder how it may be identified, found, and grasped?"

I begin each day wondering what new truth I will find in my reading and through the experiences of the day. This sense of wonderment tells me that life can be born afresh every day; and that retirement, or the final stage of life, is abundant with new possibilities—with new truths hidden in old experiences that are awaiting to be reborn if only I will take the time to reflect upon my past and consider my future. How did he say it, whomever it was: "Today is the first day of the rest of my life!" So be it.

So I enter the day ahead with my eyes wide open. How about you?

Forty-Three

Your Memory Is Part of Your Present Life!

I was faced by a significant challenge in my life this morning. The writer referred to one of the writings of Toni Morrison. In it, she is said to have described how the Mississippi River has been straightened out in places to make room for houses and livable acreage, and how occasionally the river will return to flood those places. "*Flood* is the word they use," she said, "but in fact, it is not flooding: it is remembering. Remembering where it used to be. All water has a perfect memory and is forever trying to get back to where it was."

She went on to say, "People, too, have perfect memory for some things, and one of the purposes of reviewing our own histories is to remind ourselves of where we were before we were straightened out and paved over." Personal recollection can help us to remember what we already know, and the healing properties of memory and imagination—which, of course, are blood relations—can help us to recapture our natural curves. History is a story, and the telling of stories is the doing of soul work.

The suggestion is that we need to periodically review our life to see where we have been—to see if we have continued to move in the right direction.

Greg Levoy suggests that "our past is intricately woven into our cells, and we can learn much about those cells by casting the occasional glance backward. The past tells us what has been passed on to us, and what we're attuned to because of it." He further suggests that "the past contains hints about the deeper-than-conscious goals toward which the movement of our lives is trying to take us,"—the thread, as Ira Progoff says—"that has always alternated between being visible and invisible, between surfacing and diving."

"By opening the inactive file," says Progoff, "we may discover the lost opportunities of our lives. Though some of them are dead, others are merely dormant."

Levoy writes, "We might remember the times we held off fateful encounters with the truth, avoided dealing with something that we have never been able to shake, or suffered a crisis whose message completely escaped us. We may see the times we followed the path of reason rather than intuition, the path of least resistance rather than the right way. We may remember unfinished business and decide that we can find meaning in finishing it, possibly even revelation."

Now about the challenge mentioned above. Throughout my life, as I reflect, I have been guilty of moving from one stage in my life to the next and, in the process, forgetting the individuals who were part of my life then whom I wish were still a part of my life now.

I remember a story about Catherine Marshall—the wife of the famed Presbyterian minister Peter Marshall—who, when she thought she was dying, decided to write all the people she remembered she had wronged to make amends. To set the record straight and clean up her conscience.

Is there a time in our lives when we have to stop and think about all the people in our lives with whom we have lost contact? To update ourselves and them of all that has happened to us since we parted company years ago because of disagreement or distance, and to learn something about their history? This time of research might go a long way toward making us aware of what our past has accomplished and what we might be able to do in the present and the future that will add substance to our lives. There is something about going back before we start over!

It sounds like a fun exercise: to catch up with the past, meet the present, and plan for the future! I wonder how much we have missed and need to learn about? It is like waiting for a new adventure to begin. How exciting!

Forty-Four

We Need to Try and Finish All the Stories That Are a Part of Our Lives!

As I began to write on a previous page, there is a value, or so some have suggested, for us to reexamine our past to see if we are moving in a *right direction*. I believe we need to reflect upon the stories that are a part of our past lives to reconsider our actions and our words—to see where we possibly went wrong. How many friendships or relationships did we short-circuit because of a spoken word that should have been retracted, or an action that should have been followed by an apology?

The problem that came upon me as I wrote those words is that many, if not most, of the individuals whom I seemed to have erased from my mind, in one way or another, are now gone. I can no longer communicate with them, in letter or voice, to recreate a relationship that I destroyed through my inadvertent closing of one door or another. There are so many whom I seemed to have passed by and ceased to remember. How does one make amends to people whom they passed by in the swift race we call life; individuals who played a key role in one's development and who suddenly, for what appeared to be a valid reason, were relegated to a past that has been forgotten in the present and, because they are not remembered today, will certainly be completely forgotten tomorrow?

Grey Levoy writes, "The past contains hints about the deeper-than-conscious goals toward which the movement of our lives is trying to take us. The past reminds us that we've not only risen to the challenge before and taken on daunting calls, but also, occasionally, stepped in the ring with a prizefighter and not been utterly undone, even if we haven't prevailed. It shows us what wisdom we've wrested from experience and what powers we've earned for our troubles. For many of us, the past contains the records of a diaspora, the scattering of our life's purposes and integrity, and the strewing of our priorities, the way we've wandered out of earshot of whatever is calling to us. Recollection is a way we can again remember ourselves, gather what has been dispersed, and in the process, perhaps throw off a few curses…"

As I have said, most of the people in my life who played a role in my development—professionally, socially, and otherwise—are now out of reach or have passed on. I could write a letter to each one of them and recount for them my awareness of what I did wrong, and ask for their forgiveness and for a renewal of our friendship or our relationship. Now since I do not know where they live, I probably could not send the letter, but in the writing, I could find some peace with myself. Then I could keep searching for them in the hope of one day conveying my thoughts to them as well.

I can only hope that some who might read these words will take an inventory of their own personal lives to think about whom they might have left behind—to think of those who they may have unintentionally passed by and endeavor to communicate with them in a letter, by phone, or on the internet. I only wish I had awakened to this bad habit while I still had time to satisfy my faults.

How many people do I wish I could contact just one more time to convey to them my appreciation for all that they did for me and my sorrow over what I did to them: to re-establish a contact that, even if it is not used again, is open?

In the nineteenth century, Ira Progoff describes in his writing, *At A Journal Workshop*, a group of archaeologists who discovered an ancient Egyptian tomb in which lay a portion of a tree. Embedded in the wood was a seed, which they planted to see if anything would happen. They never expected that after three thousand years, the seed would grow, but it did! Oh, the stories that could be finished if only I had taken the time and opportunity to find and rekindle their ongoing development; stories that make up my past and now impact my life, still partly unfinished…

How about the unfinished stories in your life? What do you need to do to rekindle and complete them? I wonder…

Forty-Five

We Need to Find the Core That Is at the Center of Our Lives!

N.T. Wright, a bishop of the Church of England, has this note in his book, *Simply Christian*:

> "Without God's Spirit, there is nothing we can do that will count in God's kingdom. Without God's Spirit the Church simply can't be the Church."

He is speaking of the Christian day we call Pentecost, the day Christians believe God gave his presence to the church. One would have to go to the Book of Acts to be familiar with the incident. Then he adds, "The wind and the fire and the brooding bird are given to enable the church to be the church—in other words, to enable God's people to be God's people."

It has to do with the question, "What is the core belief that guides one's life?" It goes along with a statement made in a lecture at the Ligonier Valley Study Center by Dr. R. C. Sproul: "To get the answers one needs to find, one needs to know the right questions to ask." What is the core belief in my life? What might be the core belief in your life?

What is the center of my being? For me, the question becomes, "Who is the center of my being?" My faith is what makes me whole!

My faith provides me with a place to begin every morning as I set out to live the day before me. It provides me with a beginning place with a point of reference that will enable me to understand how I want to view life: with a foundation that will explain each and every one of my actions to me and, as needed, to others!

As I sit at my desk, I read on the wall from a plaque these words of football coach Vince Lombardi: "Winning is not a sometime thing. I's an all-time thing. You don't win once in a while. You don't do things once in a while. You do them right all the time! Winning is a habit! Unfortunately, so is losing." I think what Lombardi means is that the primary focus of one's life determines the way one lives out their days.

Once again, we are pointed to the story of our lives: with how they began, with what we were taught, with what we have done with our talents, situations, and opportunities. Yes, we move from here to there. We have those moments when we lose, but these ought to be only momentary setbacks, accidents, and/or situations where we, for a moment or two, lose sight of who we are and what we want to do with our lives.

So our need is to reach out and grasp tightly that "something:" those principles that stand at the center of our living. We need to see everything in the light of that core belief. We need to rehearse its presence regularly, every morning, as we make our plans for the day as we find ourselves in one encounter or another. With it in place in the central place of our thinking, we will always be moving in the right direction.

And when we find ourselves wondering where we are and if we are doing things right, we need to stand back and look at where we are and what we are doing through that core belief that stands at the center of our being. If we lose sight of who we are and what our guiding principle is, there is nothing we can do that will count in life as far as our lives are concerned.

Forty-Six

We Need to Find and Use the Potential That We Find within Ourselves!

Think about these words of Winston Churchill:

> "There comes a special moment in everyone's life, a moment for which that person was born. That special opportunity, when he seizes it, will fulfill the mission—a mission for which he is uniquely qualified. In that moment, he finds greatness. It is his finest hour."

One wonders, have we come upon that special moment in our own lives? Or is it still out there in the future, waiting to confront us, to include us in the sweeping, ongoing development of history? Look back on all the years that have already passed. Think about all the incidents and situations that have been a part of your life. Have there been any special times when you have had to dig deep down into yourself to satisfy a particular need or confront a particular encounter? A time when you acted and felt particularly good about your action? If not, are you still looking for it?

Maybe all these years of study, work, and/or experience have yet to pay off. Perhaps your moment is still in the offing, waiting for you to get there, primed and ready to act, to do your thing in life for life!

REFLECTIONS OF A RELUCTANT RETIREE

I think that the later years in one's life, when we are not consumed by our 7:00 a.m. to 6:00 p.m. or later work lives, those times and years when we find ourselves racing from here to there and back again, doing all that needs to be done—it is *now* when we will recognize that particular moment or those special times when we can bring all of ourselves to bear on a particular need or situation that will confront us. The busyness of life may have hidden a similar situation earlier, but now, in the quiet moments of retirement and reflection, possibly now we are ready to see and act upon some opportunity, problem, or situation that presents itself to us.

As we get older, people are apt to open themselves up to us, and all of a sudden we have the time and the opportunity to show a special interest in them. All at once, we can bring the best of ourselves to bear upon someone or something that can benefit from our involvement with them or with it.

I read of a man years ago: while reading his morning newspaper, he came upon the story of a man who had been involved in an accident and was bedridden and in a coma. He decided to communicate with him through the U.S. mail. He began to write the man weekly, and sometimes more than once a week, until he received word that he had come out of his coma. He included in his epistles, words of encouragement, and hope. Sometime later, the writer heard from the victim's daughter. Her comments included one statement that truly touched him: "Your letters gave my dad hope and, I think, were largely responsible for his survival and healing. Thank you!"

While he had been working, the writer of the letters probably would not have had the time necessary to send his letters of encouragement that he now was able to compose and send. This was his moment! He found it, and he was ready to take advantage of it. How satisfied he must have been.

I would invite you to keep looking for your finest hour. Maybe it has already happened, but if it hasn't, it is still out there somewhere, someplace, waiting to happen. Maybe another opportunity will open itself up to you. It is—it will be—waiting for your response and involvement. Keep looking, and be ready!

Forty-Seven

We Can All Make a Difference in the House Where We Live!

One of the gifts that retirement brings with it is time. Time to do those things that we have always wanted to do but never had the time to do. A new vocational adventure: the development of a hobby, or the redoubling of the time we can spend on an already-adopted pastime. As I suggested in a previous writing, we have the chance now to make a difference in the worlds where we live.

Then I got to thinking. One area where we can really make a difference and can truly do something momentous is in our home. How many of us have never spent the time we ought to have spent doing things at home, around the house with our spouse and family, kids, and grandchildren?

Mark Sanborn writes in his book, *The Fred Factor*, "How would your spouse react if you demonstrated a renewed commitment to your marriage and to your relationship with her? What about your kids? One of the sadder things in life is to know someone loves us but to rarely experience their love. You can transform ordinary family interactions and events into extraordinary moments and experiences by applying what he calls "The Fred Factor" to them. The "Fred Factor" principles that he suggests we might apply, according to the author, include: Remembering that everyone makes a difference; that success is built on relationships; that you must continually create value for others, and it doesn't have to cost a penny—that you can reinvent yourself regularly! Doesn't life number 2 suggest that we point our arrows of high achievement and success inwardly, toward the environment in our home? It is something worth thinking about.

I have had a number of opportunities to preside at what couples call "a renewal of their wedding vows." It is a ceremony that gives them the opportunity to make a fresh start in their marriage. Now that does not necessarily mean that they have not been getting along and doing things right all along, or that they were on the verge of a separation and suddenly thought that a recommitment to one another is in order. Rather, it is to say that there are couples, and probably many of them, who suddenly realize that they have not been getting out of their marriage all that they intended to receive from it.

One of the realizations that comes to them, as time passes, is that they didn't have the time for each other that they had intended to give to one another on their wedding day. Now, however, they have the time. All they need to get restarted in their relationship on the right foot is to renew their commitment to one another and determine, anew, what they both want to give and receive from one another during the remaining years of their lives.

What better time is there than following our first or second retirement to determine to expend our energies and our interest on the person with whom we have been living, with whom we have had our children, and with whom we have been living out our lives? They have been looking forward to our retirement, maybe more than we have. Take a look at *The Fred Factor*'s guiding principles. Personalize them and make them a reality in your life, and do it today! In the process, give those around you—your spouse and your family—what they have been looking for and waiting for, for so many years!

FORTY-EIGHT

We Need to Remember the Past: It May Explain the Present!

When those who had lost their homes in the 1909 fire in Oakland, California, were asked by interviewers what they grabbed first on their way out the door, most of them said, "My photo albums!" We may say that the past is dead, that it's irrelevant, and that the present moment is all that matters; but it isn't true. The past is alive and well and full of pertinence. The past matters, or as someone has somewhere written, "The past is prologue!"

So why the albums? Because we want to remember who we are and how far we've come; how we lived and what was central to that life; what we've gained or lost; and who we survived or didn't. The writer Lee Abbot says, "We want to know what is in the trunks and lockers we lug forward through time: what vital secrets can be sprung to reveal."

Greg Levoy writes, "History is, above all, the story of change, and it's riddled with the unexpected—the upset decision, the sneak attack, the iceberg dead ahead, the confoundment of the elements, the unforeseen intervention." The past is vital to the future, and there's a bond between where we have been and where we are going.

My wife and I are guilty of not taking too many pictures of ourselves and our kids in their growing up years. Our children do! I don't think that we have many pictures in our storage space, though soon, after I write these words, I am going to search out all the pictures and put a label to them.

I remember visiting a lady some years ago. When she invited me into her home, she apologized for the mess we found. She had pictures everywhere. She said, "I am writing on the back of each picture who is in it and, if possible, where it might have been taken. If I don't," she said, "when I am dead and gone and my kids find these pictures in a box, they will throw them away because they won't have any sense of who the people in the pictures are, or why they might be important to them and their kids." She is gone now. I wonder if her kids paid any attention to her work. Whatever! I am going to follow in her footsteps. Hopefully, I will have enough time!

I guess what needs to happen—and again, I didn't do it myself—is kids need to ask questions. They need to fortify themselves, and eventually their children in the knowledge of the history of the family. Most of my history is gone. I will never be able to retrieve it. I know I will have to buy one of those books that ask grandparents to answer personal questions about themselves and tax their memories so that they can pass on whatever to the next generations.

The past is alive and full of pertinence. The past matters! But it has to be an informed past. We have to identify the secrets to be found in our historical lockers and pass along all that valuable information. It should never be lost!

Forty-Nine

It Is Important That We Be "a Listener" as We Travel Our Life's Road!

It was Thomas Kelly who wrote, "Lead a listening life! Order your outward life so that nothing drowns out the listening."

One of the traits that seems to have become a part of my personality as I have grown older and away from the professional life is that *I talk too much*! Possibly I have always talked too much. I would ask my wife about it, but she would be truthful; and I am not sure that I want that question answered. Anyway, today I seem to have gained a negative edge to so many things, something—so I am told—that is a part of "the old age syndrome." Things don't seem to be as they ought to be, and boy, do I let people know about it. As Kelly says, "I need to listen more and talk less."

Listening! There is so much to hear if only one can be quiet long enough to hear it. So as the years pass and I seem to have an opinion about more and more, I need to learn that I really do not have that much to say; and if I have a lot to say, I need to ask myself, *Does anybody care?*

As I have mentioned earlier, children need to ask questions—good ones and bad ones—because questions produce responses that people want to hear. So maybe I need to wait and listen to the questions that people have so as not to offer answers to questions that people have not yet asked. In other words, I need to keep my mouth shut until I have something to say that people want to hear!

I used to tell my sons while we were playing basketball, "Pass the ball two or three times before anyone shoots." It is an activity that produces teamwork and also makes sure games are not only for those who want to shoot excessively. We used to call them "pumpers," and their numbers are legion. Maybe there is validity to be found in letting people do two- or three-fourths of the talking before one enters in a response. That is, unless they are old people like ourselves who talk too much.

"Lead a listening life!" Talk less! Listen before you talk! Talk *after* you have listened. It will make for less complaining on your part and more positive conversation. I just need to listen to myself before I talk too much.

Fifty

We Need to Be a Light That Never Burns Out!

There is a wonderful little story that I think involved the author Robert Louis Stevenson. It seems that in his latter years, he was confined to a wheelchair. One evening, as he was sitting in his chair looking out of a balcony window, one of his helpers asked him what he was doing. Stevenson is said to have pointed at the man who was lighting the lamps on the street below, and said, "I am watching the lamplighter punch holes in the darkness."

What an important job or opportunity! In a world where there is so much stress and strain, so much depression and death, to be able to see someone, or to yourself, punch some holes of light into the darkness of another's life—what a wonderful thing that could and would be. We all need to have a little bit of hope in our lives, and how blessed we are when someone lights that light in our lives.

It could be the greeter at the local Walmart. It could be someone who offers us a word of encouragement when we are confronting the death of a loved one, or enduring a "down moment" in our job. It could be a hand on our shoulder in a doctor's office, or in a hospital waiting room, or in any other difficult time or place in our lives. Certainly, there are many such times or situations in most of our lives.

Or we could be the giver of hope and encouragement. We, ourselves, could be a lamplighter. As we walk through our lives, particularly in our later years, we can be both the receiver and/or the giver of some light! We certainly have the time. We only need to make some effort. Just imagine the opportunity to lift up someone else's spirit, offering a word of encouragement or just our presence when someone is walking through a dark moment.

There are some people who bring light into any room they enter. We all know such people. Individuals who are so in touch with their own lives that they do not need to draw attention to themselves but can give it to anyone of us. We can be those kind of people out there on life's road, wherever we are…

I was taking my daily walk in our local mall. I chanced upon a woman who, she said, had just buried her mother. Since we were longtime friends, she stopped me and seemed just to want to talk. We did so for some time. When we parted, she seemed to be lighter on her feet. She had expended some of her grief, and it put a bounce back into her step. All it took on my part was a little bit of time, and certainly, at this point in my life, I have the time to give. Why not to someone else?

We need to put a smile on our face and some bounce in our step and to be aware of the needs of the people around us. Just a smile, but more often a word of encouragement and hope: and the world can be a better place for all of us.

Enter the journey! Share your gifts! Experience the joy of passing on your words of hope and encouragement. Share a part of your life! We will all be the better for it!

All it will take is a little bit of our time! Just a *little bit* of it!

Fifty-One

We Are All in Need of Some Self-Discipline!

Early in his classic writing, *The Road Less Traveled*, M. Scott Peck wrote: "Once we truly know that life is difficult, once we truly understand and accept it, then life is no longer difficult." Further down the page, he adds, "Life is a series of problems," and then he shares his solution. "Discipline is the best set of tools we require to solve life's problems."

The presumption is that in the words of Steven Covey, "We need to be proactive in our approach to life." We need to know where we are going (vision) and how we want to get there (discipline). The problems of which he speaks are the bumps in the road, as we move from *here* to *there*.

As I have to constantly remind myself, "Vision is the vehicle that moves me from where I am to where I am going to be or want to be." The problem is, I do not know where I want to be. I do not know how I want to spend the remainder of the time that I have left in this life. Nobody can tell me where I should go, and I have a difficult time telling myself where I want to go. Peck tells me, if this is my problem, that I have to create a discipline to get me somewhere. I have suggested, in previous reflections, that as far as I understand it, I have to create a discipline that will prepare me to go where life will direct me. I have limited opportunities or roads on which to walk, so I have to carefully look at who I am and what road I ought to take.

Disciplines do not have to be difficult or involved. They just have to keep me in tune so that when life calls, I am ready to respond.

So I fashion a discipline. I must ask myself how I will use particular periods of my time, and then how the other time periods, the time remaining, ought to be utilized. Now I am a person that is used to having an organization with which to work and personnel who can share with me in the journey. Now in this latter period of my life, other personnel are not available. Now I am moving along life's way *alone*. So if I am going to undertake one project or another, I have to reach out to gather together the appropriate personnel to help me accomplish any task that I wish to tackle.

Consequently, I must continue to hone the tools that I have put in my tool belt and wait. Always, there is time available to consider what I am doing and how well I am doing it. Following the discipline that I have already adopted, all I can do is wait with open eyes and ears! I wonder what lies ahead of me. How about you?

FIFTY-TWO

We Need Help as We Deal with Life's Difficulties!

I recently picked up a book on a sale table in one of the bookstores that I visit. It was written by Denis Waitley and entitled, *Empires of the Mind: Lessons to Lead and Succeed in a Knowledge Based World*! It was written away back in 1995, so I am sure that the statistics quoted are now even larger than as printed, as our population has grown and our attitude toward education continues to diminish.

Waitley was, and undoubtedly continues to be, a recognized leader in the area of leadership development. Speaking about the present century, the twenty-first, Waitley writes, "We are about to enter a new century of unprecedented human growth and development. We must reexamine and reevaluate the way we think and the way we respond to life's daily challenges, in which will be a time of even more astonishing change. We need a fresh, enduring strategy for viewing our potential and mapping our goals—goals that are worthwhile, believable, and achievable."

Waitley concerned himself about the demands of continuing change that now confront the worlds in which we live. Education for this, the twenty-first century, is gained, of course, in the classroom but beyond and even more so in the environs of one's reading. He presents a significant fact, perhaps more advanced today than at the time of his writing: "Fewer than ten percent of us buy and read non-fiction books." Then he adds this observation: "Most people prefer to do just enough to get by. Reading and learning is too much like hard work. They'd rather get home that get ahead."

He says, "People would increase their learning and earning power immeasurably by spending half as much time reading as they waste gaping at television." And "not long ago, what you learned in school was largely all you needed to learn. You could rely on that knowledge for the rest of your life. This is no longer true. Your formal education has a very short shelf life."

He concludes: "Lifelong learning, once a luxury for the few, has become absolutely vital to continued success."

Thinking back to the words of M. Scott Peck, reading then becomes one of the significant disciplines as we face and prepare for life, even and more so in the later times of life. If the average individual spent as much time reading as they do gaping at their television screen, how much wiser and up to date might we become? I mean, nonfiction reading. So as the years pass by, a weekly visit to the library or the bookseller certainly will assist us as we continue to deal with the problems that life sends our way, and that we are called upon to deal with regularly. "Lifelong learning…has become absolutely vital!"

Fifty-Three

We Need to Understand That a Good Discipline Takes Time to Develop!

"Good discipline takes time!" So writes M. Scott Peck as he speaks of parental relations with their children in his book, *The Road Less Traveled*. I am going to take the privilege of taking his words out of their literary context and apply them to almost any circumstance in life. "Good discipline takes time to develop!"

Whether it has to do with the time a child takes to absorb the teaching of its parents, or the patience a parent must muster while they wait for a child or children to catch on to the lessons they are trying to teach them—time is required for a discipline to grow into the habits that are being formed.

Yes, a discipline takes time to develop, and even more time is required when it comes to the development of a personal discipline. I came across another statement, in another reading, that suggested, "In a world in which working with people is essential, it also means developing your understanding of yourself and others. To know oneself means," as the Oracle of Delphi suggests, "to be aware not only of one's potential but also of one's personal expectations." The issue becomes "What do I do with myself, and how will that impact on the world in which I live?" And furthermore, how will it affect my expectations of other people.

I sit in my own presence from day-to-day, looking at the day and at the time, wondering what would be the most advantageous way for me to use my time and my effort. As the years pass by—all too quickly, I might add—I continue to realize that being satisfied with my use of my own time is the most important commodity in a successful life. I have no one to answer to: I have to answer only to myself and to my God. If life is a mystery, now, it is only a mystery because the future is impenetrable. And I use that word not because I don't know what tomorrow might hold in store for me, but because there are no assumptions or schedules that will, in any way, help me to make those determinations.

With no demands and no expectations, there is a tendency to put off until tomorrow anything and everything. There is *always* tomorrow, and tomorrow is free and open; no demands, etc. So the discipline needed is to create a timeline and to focus on meeting a series of self-created things to do. Satisfaction is then found in crossing off those tasks one by one, and when they have all been completed to say, "I have met the demands that list has put on me," it is time to create another list.

However, to do that means creating a discipline of time management. The temptation is to casually move into each day and its anticipations, and that means that adjustments will have to be made in the formulation of one's discipline. "That will wait until tomorrow…" Right?

Good discipline takes time! However, time is of the essence, so one's time must be put at the disposal of a discipline. I remember sitting at a meeting with someone who had just gone through a time-management course. She had a large notebook that was the essence of the program. Her comment, however, as it comes back to me, at that moment was, "I have to plan in the evening what I am going to do the next day." Well, that is what time management is all about, and that is something that one must plant in the basic core of one's life. Chapter and paragraph must be determined prior to opening the book of a new day. If good discipline takes time, one must be aware of the fact that there is only so much time. Yes, friend, there is only so much time, and it is a wasting!

Fifty-Four

We Need to Realize That It Takes Time to Deal with the Challenges That Life Places Before Us!

In the aforementioned book, *Empires of the Mind*, Denis Waitley writes:

> "Start thinking of yourself as a service company with a single employee." Then, "You're the CEO who must have the vision to set your goals and allocate your resources. Since your primary concern is ensuring your viability in the marketplace, you must think strategically in every decision. This mindset of being responsible for your own future used to be critical only to the self-employed, but it has become essential for us all. For today's typical Americans are no longer one-career people. Most will have five separate careers in their lifetimes."

At this particular moment in time, as I stand before, what I anticipate will be the final career of my lifetime; I feel compelled to consider the resources that I have marshaled by birth, education, and experience, and determine how I can best use them to find satisfaction and fulfillment during the remaining years of my life. There are probably more resources available than I give myself credit for possessing. One of my primary needs, as suggested in the previous writing, is to find the patience to assess the situations that are in front of me and then determine how I can bring my limited abilities to bear upon them.

M. Scott Peck speaks of having limited mechanical ability. My family tells me that I am technologically challenged as well. The reasons are the same. Not the lack of ability, necessarily, but the unwillingness, on my part, to take the time to see any one task through to its completion. At this point in time, I hate to read directions. In fact, I have never liked to read directions. It is so much easier to find someone else to do one or another of the tasks that confront me.

Peck writes that he came across a neighbor who was repairing his lawn mower. His comment to the neighbor was, "Boy, I sure admire you. I've never been able to fix those kinds of things, or do anything like that."

The neighbor is reported to have shot back, without a moment's hesitation, "That's because you don't take the time."

Peck continues, "I resumed my walk, somehow disquieted by the gurulike simplicity, spontaneity, and defensiveness of his response." He then asked himself the question, "You don't suppose he could have been right, do you?"

Later in his account, he writes that he was faced with a situation similar to the one that had confronted his neighbor. Remembering the reprimand, he writes that he took the time to survey the situation, and Hallelujah, he was able to find within himself the mechanical ability to satisfy the problem and reap the person's appreciation. It just demanded that he apply his patience to the situation at hand.

"That's because you don't take the time!" Upon the reexamination of my life, I have to admit that that statement is a truism which I need to consider. It is a major problem for me. Remember, I don't read directions! I do not like to do things on my own if I can, at all, help it. If I can receive the benefits of someone else's reading, I will. When my wife says, "Read this or that," I say, "What did it say." She usually responds in exasperation, "Just read it!" Sometimes I do, and sometimes I don't. I call my request "delegation," and is that not what a CEO ought to do?

The same fact holds true when it comes to household tasks that require some research and development on my part. My wife's order, "Just do it!" However, I know there is someone out there who can do it easier and better than I can. I just know it. So I will go and search them out! There is a problem here: that is, my spouse does not appreciate the time interval. She, of course, just needs to be patient.

I woke up this morning to the realization that some of the disciplines that I need to incorporate or reincorporate into my life are right in front of me. The primary need is to ascertain what they are and how I can use them.

"Discipline!" "Discipline!" "Discipline!" "That's because you don't take the time." This is where I am! This is where I think I want to be! The question is, "How will I get from here to there?" I think—in fact, I know—that I need to take the time to consider each situation that confronts me and determine how I can deal with it personally. The word then becomes *patient self-improvement*!

"That's because you don't take the time!" Yikes!

FIFTY-FIVE

We Need to Deal with Today's Problems Today!

"Don't put off until tomorrow what you can do today!" Or in the words of a man who is much wiser than I am or will ever be: "We cannot solve life's problems except by solving them." Sounds like a Yogi Berra Ism, but it is not. In any event, there is a lot of wisdom in that statement: something worth thinking about.

How many times have we placed a decision on hold and then found that when we are ready to make it, it has already been made for us? Sometimes to our advantage; sometimes, sadly, to our disadvantage. Then we reminisce, "Why didn't I decide to do or not to do it sooner? How has our life been changed or redirected because we decided to put off until tomorrow or next week or next month something we should have done much sooner? How many times have we put off making a decision until it was too late?

The problem with living in the second half of one's life is, that now, today, we don't have any real assurance to believe that we will be around tomorrow to make a decision that we don't seem to want to make today. Age and the progressive state of our health suggests that tomorrow might never come, and if it does, we might not be in a position to have a choice relative to what we shall do or where we shall go!

We buy some flowers to plant in our yard, but we decide to put them into the ground or planter tomorrow and not today. Then some situation or event transpires, and the option is no longer available to us. In the meanwhile, they die, and someone else throws them away; and that special spot, for which we intended them, remains bleak and unattended.

A word of advice to you, but most particularly to me. Make a list! One by one, list the situations and/or problems that have confronted you and continue to face you in your living. Personal? Professional? Social? Cultural? I would venture to say that many of the unsolved situations or problems that exist today in my life are the same ones that afflicted my life twenty, thirty, forty, or even sixty-five years ago in one size or form or another. The continue to be on my To Do list! How about you? How many times have we said, "I will deal with it or that tomorrow!" Well, like it or not, tomorrow is here today!

We ask ourselves, "What are they? Why do these situations and/or problems continue to afflict me?" Answer: because we have never determined to confront and solve them!

First, of course, the list! Some things are trivial. Get the windshield on my car fixed! Have the rear bumper of the car attended to! Change the light bulb in the bedroom! Do an inventory of my wardrobe. What needs to be discarded? Replaced?

Others are likely to be more important. Put my will and my insurance papers in an appropriate place, and tell my spouse where that might be. Maybe the will needs to be updated! How about a power of attorney? Are our living wills available to the members of our family who might have to use them?

At this point, I am sure that many of the problems and situations that have traveled with me through the years don't make much difference anymore. Yet maybe upon reflection, they demand some action. In any event, I will list them, and if they can be solved, I will solve them! Even, I might add, even if that means determining *not* to do something anymore.

We cannot solve life's problems except by solving them!

Fifty-Six

We Need to Have Some Quiet Times so We Can Hear What Our Lives Are Trying to Tell Us!

In the midst of his book of daily meditations entitled, *Listening to Your Life*, Frederick Buechner writes, "God speaks to us. I would say much more often than we realize or that we choose to realize. Before the sun sets every evening, he speaks to each one of us in an intensely personal and unmistakable way. His message is not written out in starlight which, in the long run, would make no difference. Rather, it is written out for each of us in the humdrum helter-skelter events of each day. It is a message that, in the long run, might just make all the difference."

Then he adds, "I suspect that, that maybe God speaks to us more clearly through his silence, his absence, so that we know him best through our missing him."

He also speaks to us about ourselves, about what he wants us to do, and what he wants us to become; and this is the area where I believe we know much more about him than we admit, even to ourselves. It is on that inner level that people hear God, even if they do not believe in him.

And then, "Our days are full of nonsense, and yet not, because it is precisely into the nonsense of our days that God speaks to us words of great significance. Not words that are written in the stars, but words that are written into the raw stuff and nonsense of our days, which are not nonsense. God speaks to us in the midst of them. And the words that he says to each one of us differently are: 'be brave,' 'be merciful,' 'feed my lambs,' 'press on toward the goal.'"

The suggestion seems to be that whether we know it or not, or believe it or not, God is *always* in the process of speaking to us. Our only task, and it is one we do not assume for ourselves, is to pick up what he has to say in the very midst of the noise that we have inflicted on our lives. God knows where he wants us to go and what he wants us to do and what he wants us to be, but we are so busy trying to decipher these things for ourselves that we do not hear his voice. It is only by means of an open ear, mind, and heart that we ever reach that point where we can understand what God's vision for us really is. Many of us never come to grips with that vision; never see it; never fulfill it. And probably, unhappiness descends upon us and gets a grip on us because of our inattentiveness. Sometimes we never free ourselves from its grip and garner what God really has in store for us.

We interject our will on ourselves and never let God have his way. How sad! How very sad! To think that his message is a mere heartbeat away, hidden from us by some words that we think we have to speak or write. We have to be more quiet, to be silent, to allow God to speak to us out of the shadows. I wonder? Can I be quiet enough to hear what God has to say to me? I really wonder? I really wonder if I can be quiet enough to hear God's voice—the still small voice that sought to speak to Elijah. I hope to get to hear what God is trying to say to me before I go to sleep, before he has to tell me what he wants me to hear, face-to-face, in the brightness of the eternal morning light. If I have to wait that long, what will I have missed?

FIFTY-SEVEN

Each One of Us has Our Own "Road Less Traveled!"

The second reading of a book always gives us the opportunity to make some new discoveries! Such has been the case with my rereading of M. Scott Peck's work, *The Road Less Traveled*. The writing has been reintroduced to me by the minister at the church where we worship.

Peck remarks, "The life of wisdom must be a life of contemplation combined with action." Now the "examination of the world without is never as personally painful as the examination of the world within, and it is certainly because of the pain involved in a life of genuine self-examination that the majority of us steer away from." Frankly, I am not sure we steer away from it so much as we don't take the time to look within ourselves in the midst of the hurry and scurry of our busy lives.

Anyway, Peck continues, "The only way that we can be certain that our map of reality is valid is to expose it to the criticism and challenge of other map makers," or in other words, compare our lives to the lives of other individuals who are living in a similar area and/or moving in the same type of circle in which we are moving.

Think about it now. We have the opportunity to read the biographical and autobiographical records not only of famous individuals but also of people like us who have walked or are walking on the same path we have determined to walk and in the same direction we seem to be going.

"The map!" It will help us to find our own "road less traveled." *Less traveled* because we are the first to walk down its lonely way, at least as far as we know. *Lonely* because we are the only one's putting our feet to its path. Yes, we may cross other roads, including the paths of other people who are on their own separate journey, and even walk with them for a while. However, for the most part, our road is one we walk by ourselves always, I might add, in the company of the ever-present God!

I guess my problem is, as it may be for you and for others, the whole act of contemplation. I find it hard to be still. I can do it, yes, but it ain't easy. It is a daily struggle for me, but I keep working at it. One way to accomplish this undertaking, although some might not call it an act of contemplation, is to write down the reflections that dawn upon us while we are silently thinking our way through our past and present lives. In those seconds, minutes, and hours, ideas come to mind; faults of the past come to the surface, and as they do and we write them down for later consideration, we can later seek to reinvent ourselves to satisfy their demands.

As we do this, our lives change. They move in one direction and then in another. The problem is, as with problems that might dot a "prayer list," when we seem to have them under control, suddenly they reappear, and we have to deal with them all over again. I suspect that is one of the primary activities of our lives; that is, dealing with the same problems over and over again as they present themselves to us, as if for the first time.

Always then, reflection is my need: contemplation is my challenge and the continuing exposure of my life to the light of life; my primary responsibility. I read recently, and my source has disappeared onto one of the bookshelves in my study, of a man who wrote his autobiography when he had retired and reached the age of seventy. Twenty years later, when he had reached the age of ninety, he realized he had to write an epilogue to his earlier thoughts.

The conclusion: It is never too late to reflect. Contemplation is the lifeblood of an active and resourceful journey. So what are my—are your—problems today? Which one do I—do you—tackle first? I wonder...

Fifty-Eight

Time Is One of Life's Most Important Commodities!

Some years ago now, an aerial photograph was made of the Statue of Liberty. The picture is said to have revealed the extraordinary detail that was designed into the top of the statue's head by the sculptor Frederick August Bartholdi. Now please remember, the statue was designed in the 1870s, long before the invention of the airplane and the sculptor had no reason to suspect that those details would ever be seen by anyone other than some high-flying seagulls. However, it is reported that Bartholdi was motivated from within to pursue excellence in all his work. So he refused to cut corners on his masterpiece. As he wrote, "Maybe no one else would know, but I will know." That was motivation enough for him to give his attention to every detail of this great work of art.

Years later, Oscar Hammerstein II had this to say, following his viewing of the aerial photograph: "When you are creating a work of art or another kind of work, finish the job perfectly. You never know when someone will fly over your work and find you out."

Life is one of those works of art. Yes, people can catch a glimpse of our work by surveying our birth certificate and the other pieces of paper we accumulated during our intellectual and marketplace experiences. They can read our diaries and interview our family, coworkers, friends, and neighbors. But what about all the silent, unrecorded minutes, hours, and years? I would venture to say that we spend more time by ourselves than with others, times not open to review. Consequently, can we not say that only we, ourselves, can measure our ultimate accomplishments? That only we, ourselves, can decide whether or not we did or did not do the most with our time?

Who can speak to how wisely we used our time of what we did for the betterment of life in general? We have so much private time to invest or to waste. Generally, our families will be very gentle in assessing what we did with those years. They are very forgiving and probably don't really give a damn about what we said or did. But we ought to.

We can stand or sit or lie in our bed at the end of each day and assess our accomplishments, and we are the only ones who can do so. We can seek forgiveness for our oversights. We can seek forgiveness from people whom we have offended: for jobs not finished, for promises not kept. Most of them, in our later years, were probably unnoticed any way.

But as to the satisfaction of all the time and opportunity that continues to be ours as the years march by, who is to be the judge? Well, Bartholdi has an answer. "We are!" So we have the task of assessing how we are doing with the gift we call life. God will also have a hand in it, but he, too, has allowed us the chance to determine how we spend our time. If we don't hurt others, if we do what is right and good, if we live according to the rules, God will be all right with that. Right?

We have the responsibility to wisely use our time, to satisfy the goals we have set for ourselves, to motivate ourselves to do what we are capable of doing. And what will that be?

Fifty-Nine

There Is Something to Be Said for Feeling a Sense of "Self-Accomplishment!"

The other day, I came across two separate sentences that seemed to fly in the face of each other. First these words of Denis Waitley: "The first step toward shaping your personal culture is launching a consciously planned excellence program to empower yourself." Now there are additional words in the sentence, but they relate what you do to those with whom you work, and I am beyond that point in my life.

The second sentence comes from the pen of M. Scott Peck: "We must be attracted, invested, and committed to an object outside of ourselves, beyond the boundaries of self. Psychiatrists call this process of attraction an investment and commitment 'cathexis,' and say that we 'cathect' the beloved subject." The one speaks of living life from the inside out, and the other of living from the outside in. Peck speaks of a man who is literally obsessed with his garden, who ultimately incorporates the garden into himself and the self into the garden. The garden then becomes an enlargement of his self.

Frankly, I consider Waitley's idea more appealing because it is easier to understand, and the two ideas end up on the same page anyway. The garden becomes the result of one's obsession; the proof of one's desire for excellence. I have done the garden thing, but it soon disappears in the fall to the ravages of the cold, snow, and winter. My obsession is more immediate. I am concerned with a personal discipline that will result in the accomplishment of something more cerebral.

Think again with me about Waitley's thesis: "The first step toward shaping your personal culture is launching a consciously planned excellence program to empower yourself." My accomplishments have always been centered on what appears on a written or printed page: the desire to explain one's thought, aspirations, and about lessons learned from others and even from myself.

I think that I have captured my program of excellence in a schedule that is particularly appropriate to myself. Everyone has their own goal and, hence, their own program. Some of our new cultures are visible; some are invisible. The gardener's aspirations are seen in the beauty of nature: in his or her relationship with the growing process. My aspirations are more inward, and the results of my program are to be found on this and other pages. What do I think? What does that mean? What can it mean?

There is a certain satisfaction to be found in doing something that will last; something that people will see and appreciate. I have moved beyond that too. Today my accomplishments are more "person-oriented." By "person-oriented," I mean that they are things that I can see and, likely, others can't.

My personally planned program toward excellence is one that only I can see. "You read too much," is what some say. But I am happy reading—let me alone! My sense of accomplishment is found today in finding new thoughts and thinking them through. Taking statements like the two mentioned above and making them my own because I can add new thoughts and twists to them.

In the latter years of one's life, satisfying one's inner needs goes a long way toward satisfying one's life needs. So each one of us has to decide what we want to accomplish, whether we want to build from the core outward or do something out there and let it take hold on the inside of us.

Sixty

Satisfaction Comes in Many Sizes and Shapes!

It is amazing how many things we read from day to day that remind us of things that we read at another time and in another place, perhaps in the long ago. The other day, I came across this statement: "I read somewhere that if we were to spend two hours a day doing something that we choose to do that makes us happy, within five years, we can become an expert at it."

The statement awakened my mind to a story that I read years ago; I think in *Reader's Digest* magazine. It was written by or about Crawford Greenawalt who, at the time, I believe, was the president and CEO of the DuPont Corporation.

During his early years, Greenawalt developed an interest in butterflies. Captured by the subject, he determined to spend an hour each day reading on the subject He never stopped. For years and years, he would dedicate an hour every day, even in the midst of a very busy corporate routine, to the study of butterflies.

By the time he had reached the pinnacle of the corporate world, he had also become an expert on the subject of butterflies. Scholars from around the world would call him for his opinion about or his counsel on one matter or another that related to the butterfly. I suspect that one of his peers or another shook their head in disbelief when he talked about his passion and the investment of his time in it.

I believe it was the mother of the actress Katherine Hepburn who advised her, "If you always do what interests you, at least one person is pleased."

It was Marcus Aurelius who concluded, "Very little is needed to make a happy life."

The thought that engendered this writing and the several quotes listed above came from a writing of Alexandra Stoddard, which she entitled, *You Are Your Choices*. In it, she tells the story of a missionary family by the name of Donnelly that she met in Madras, India. The Donnelly's told her, "When we have our favorite books, fresh flowers, meaningful work, and the companionship of each other, this is all we need to be happy." How many people who are unhappy are but one thought away from real happiness?

What will it take to make you happy? Now this is not to say that you are not already happy. However, it is to suggest that we need to take some time to reflect upon our life and our lifestyle to determine whether or not we have overlooked some past dream or aspiration that, when we are near the end of our days, will surface and tell us, "If only you had done this or that, your life would have gained a sense of completeness about it!" Why didn't you do it? Anne Lamott writes, "Your problem is how you are going to spend this one odd and precious life you have been issued. Whether you are going to taste it, enjoy it and find out the truth about who you are."

I guess today I want you to feel a little bit uncomfortable. I want you to reflect on what you haven't done in your life that tomorrow you will wish you had done. Lamott quotes these words of Breaker Morant, "You have to live every day as if it's your last, because one of these days, you're bound to be right."

So find a lawn chair under the tree in your backyard or on your deck. Lie back in your bed, or on the couch in your family room. Find someplace where you can be comfortable with yourself, and let some of your abandoned thoughts come to the top of your mind. I bet that you will discover that deep down, somewhere in there, there is something that is just itching to be reborn, nurtured, and developed. It might be something that you can accomplish in one day or in one week. Or it might be something that will take the rest of your lifetime to satisfy. But then, what else do you have to do but do it?

Sixty-One

We All Need to Create and Follow an Adventure Map!

"The more clearly we see the reality of the world, the better equipped we will be to deal with the world. The less clearly we see the reality of the world, the more our minds are befuddled by falsehood, misperceptions, and illusions—the less able we will be to determine correct courses for action and make wise decisions. Our view of reality is like a map with which to negotiate the terrain of life. If the map is true and accurate, we will generally know where we are, and if we have decided where we want to go, we will generally know how to get there. If the map is false and inaccurate, we will generally be lost."

Then these words, "The more effort we make to appreciate and perceive reality, the larger and more accurate our maps will be." However, so the writer presumes, "By the end of middle age, most people have given up the effort. Only a relative and fortunate few continue until the moment of death, exploring the mystery of reality, ever enlarging and refining and redefining their understanding of the world and what is true." And then this conclusion, "If our maps are to be accurate, we have to continually review them."

The function of these daily reflections, I hope, is to help us to be continually involved in the revision of our life's maps. The demand is to keep on keeping on! The desire is to keep reflecting on what one reads, sees, and hears, and apply those insights into one's daily experience of life.

The map is the guideline one may use to plot where one is and where one is going. The only individual concern is, "Where do I want to go?"

The world is changing fast! Agreed? Faster than I am able to run. I can only reflect today on what I learned yesterday and put it in the context of what I am experiencing in the here and now. Certainly, there are side trips. We go off on a side road or tangent, realize it is not where we want to be, go back to the main road, and keep on moving on. I guess, if we were fixed in our attention, if we continually knew who we are and where we really want to go in the remaining years of our lives, the journey would be uneventful. But I am not sure we all know? Some of us do, but most of us don't. So being befuddled is an experience that each of us must endure. It is the prelude to knowing, but knowing is a moving target. So though we are sometimes lost, if we are diligent in our thinking, we are at least moving in the right direction.

We need an adventure map! No matter where we are today, we need a map. In fact, where we are today might be better explained to us and others by working backward to our first point of remembrance. The biblical Israelites moved back to the beginning in the Genesis account after they had experienced the freedom brought to them through their Exodus experience. Genesis was composed to make themselves and the world aware of their origins. So all the material from Genesis 1 through Exodus 15 seeks to bring them up to speed in their historical and religious adventures.

And so with us, backtracking will help us to determine how we got where we are, and then our task is to plot out where we think we want to go or end up. Then we can begin to make the changes that will develop as we move on in our adventure. I think it is an exercise worthy of a try!

Sixty-Two

Many of Us Can Have a "Last Hurrah!"

During the last number of years—that is, early in the twenty-first century—filmgoers were treated to a number of movies that chronicled the fictitious adventures of several grumpy old men. As I understand it, many of us who reach retirement age and beyond become very critical of the society that is developing around us. We seem ready and able, without being asked, to offer our criticisms and our advice to others on how to right the perceived wrongs that come to our attention. We presume to believe that we see and know more than our younger counterparts who will, in the end, have to do the heavy lifting. Age seems to give us the ability to see how to set the society, in which live, on a new course and, as far as we are able to determine, in a new and better direction.

    Now we do this in spite of the fact that as older adults, we need to be mindful of the fact that it is too easy to find fault with what is going on around us. What we have to also remember is that we are the ones who created the society in which we find ourselves and with which we are finding fault. However, and this is a big word, *however*, there are things that we have brought to pass that need to be revisited and reinvented. The problem is, it takes a lot to get us moving. Too many of us are ready to sit back and complain and then let the younger generations do what needs to be done in spite of the fact that they were not the culprits that got us into the mess in which we find ourselves in the first place.

REFLECTIONS OF A RELUCTANT RETIREE

The need is for us, those of us who have been around for a long time, to see what is wrong and make every effort to correct the problems or situations before we leave this grand orb. The problem is, we have to be irritated by a circumstance or situation to the point where we want to do something about it: people today might call that moment "a tipping point."

This thought came to mind while I was reading a book by a Chicago area minister by the name of Bill Hybels. He calls the feeling that we find afflicting us, in those or these moments, "a holy discontent." As he writes, "Holy discontent can overtake you in an instant. You're going about your business, doing life as usual, when suddenly something happens that awakens your awareness and jolts your soul. A heartbreaking personal experience, a national calamity, an infuriating injustice to someone close to you—whatever it is, you can't take it lying down. You've got to do something." (The book is a good read!)

The analogy that he uses points us to a cartoon character that I remember from my childhood movie-going days, in black and white, on the screen of our local theater. Do you remember Popeye the Sailor Man? You will remember he had a girlfriend by the name of Olive Oyl and a perennial nemesis by the name of Bluto. In the series of cartoons that continue today, whenever Olive Oyl got into trouble, or Bluto created a situation that threatened the world in which he lived, Popeye would blurt out the words that many of us will always remember: "That's all I can stands, and I can't stands no more." Out would come a can of spinach which he would swallow in one lump and, with the strength it would give him, *he would save the day!*

Hybels's word of wisdom is this: "I believe the motivating reason why millions of people choose to do good in the world around them is because there is something wrong in that world."

When grumpy old men reach a tipping point, the Popeye within them materializes, almost before they know it. So watch out, world!

I have many a friend who has ripped open a can of spinach and digested it through their pipeline. They have initiated such programs as a local Habitat for Humanity Program, revived Cub and

Boy Scout troops, revitalized or helped to create one community project or another, entered politics because they felt a need to be a change agent—you probably can name friends like that as well. The point is, the problems that face us in this world of ours, of our own making or because one situation or another just went bad, demand to be addressed; and, friends, many of us have the ability—fiscally, mentally, or physically—to address them.

What is the directive we need to hear? "Don't just sit there. Do SOMETHING!" Well?

Sixty-Three

On the Joy of Starting Out All over Again!

In reflecting upon her separation from a vocation as a serving Episcopal priest and her impending change of activities, because of it, Barbara Taylor Brown offers us this thought:

> "The week after I left church, I was back on the floor again. For years, I had kept hoping the intimacy with God would blossom as soon as I got everything done, got everyone settled, and got my environment just right and my calendar cleared. I counted on it to come as a reward for how hard I had worked, or at least as the built-in consequence of a life of service, but when I managed to meet all of my conditions for a day or two, I was so exhausted from the effort that I could not keep my eyes open. Slumber spiritually took over, and when I woke up, I was right back where I started with miles to go toward the home I never quite reached."

She learned that life number 2 is more difficult to come by and plan for than life number 1. In the first life, one has their youth and their dreams and some determined goals and aspirations. In the second life, in a sense, each one of those things is gone. For Taylor, this was a midlife struggle, as it is for many, as they assume a second career or reach a new starting point during journey number 1. Their number is legion—or should I say, *our* number is legion! Youth, at least of the body, is gone. The dreams of tomorrow are still clouded in the morning sky, and the determined goals and aspirations, if not already satisfied, are no longer there.

It is the same old story again and again. Living life number 2 has no timeline, no guidelines; and if there are aspirations and dreams, they have to be refined and given form. This is what takes a long time. This is what is taking a long time.

Start overs are difficult. There are many of them. They take up many mornings, many days, maybe many months, possibly a few years. Trying to get into a rhythm where there is no beat to live by takes time. And if one is somewhat undisciplined, there is another handicap to be overcome. When one's life is scheduled by *to-do* things and lists—when they are gone and the luxury of time on your hands is available—discipline is a whole new activity. Laziness is the hazard that some will have to overcome. "I can do it tomorrow," is another…

Yet the excitement of *tomorrow* is there. "I have all this time. I just have to decide how to invest it!" These thoughts have a wonderful ring to them!

Brown's point is that the things that she was looking for, though they are out there, have to be worked for and settled into. There are no rewards! Yesterday is gone forever. Tomorrow is waiting for you, but you will have to find some new companions, have some new expectations, and realize that the future is in the planning mode. And the planning mode might take—well, maybe not forever, but certainly a long time to create and enjoy.

It is called *starting over*! And it can be a delight! It is a delight! If you are up to it…

Sixty-Four

We Can All Make a Difference in the Worlds Where We Live!

If we have maintained the enthusiasm of our youth, if we continue to be consumed by the challenges and struggles that face our worlds, if we have not lost our sense of optimism and still believe that there are possibilities inherent in us that the world can use, then these words of Mark Sanborn in his book, *The Fred Factor*, are for us.

Sanborn writes, "To admit that you begin the day planning to change the world certainly sounds grandiose, maybe even delusional. Yet I believe that you can change the world every day, whether you intend to or not. Often it only takes a small act to make a difference."

You can change the world of your spouse and/or kids depending on how you interact with them before you leave your home, or while you are visiting in their home. A little extra time or attention or a tender moment of affection changes their world that day, or any day, for that matter. It should remind you of what is really important in this busy world of ours.

Now this is not to say that your actions will affect any dramatic changes in the world. As Sanborn writes, "They will not alter the course of world affairs or bring about a cure for AIDS. However, who's to say that these little changes don't have a cumulative, profound effect in the lives of others and, ultimately, in your own life?"

Then he concludes this thought with these words: "To make a difference means affecting another person, group or situation. It is nearly impossible to remain neutral as you journey through each day. Paying attention to others, giving them the response that they deserve, and politely serving them makes a positive difference."

I read the story of a business type who was running to catch a train home. As he ran down the ramp from the station, he bumped into a little boy whom he had not seen in his hurry to catch the departing train. The lad, who was carrying an armful of toys, was waiting impatiently with his mother for their train number to be called. The toys he was carrying flew all over the place.

The businessman stopped for a minute to collect himself and then started again, running for the train. However, as he looked back at the young child, he saw tears begin to well up in the boy's eyes. So he sighed, went back to where the youngster was standing, put down his briefcase, and began to help pick up the scattered toys and hand them to the boy one by one as his train pulled out of the station.

When the boy had all his toys once again in his arms, he looked at the man and said, "Sir, are you Jesus?" Well, you know, at that moment in time, that is exactly who he was to that little boy.

You know, there is a vast world out there outside the boundaries of our home and property, waiting to be touched by interested people like you and me. Maybe, in times past, we did not take the time to stoop down and help to put someone else's world back together again; but now, today, I would guess we have the time or could take the time to do it. All we have to know and remember is, that in the midst of the second half of our lives, in our retirement years, that we still have the opportunity to be a difference maker. "True difference-making can't be delegated. It's up to us to take action."

What kind of a difference maker will you make in your world today?

Sixty-Five

How You Can Continue to be Successful!

I chanced upon a quotation of Ralph Waldo Emerson the other day that I think is worth remembering. He wrote: "The purpose of life is not to be happy. It is to be useful, to be honorable, to be compassionate, to have it make some difference that you have lived and lived well."

It has been written that individuals who want to get the most out of their lives live with this philosophy. They are always striving to give meaning to their lives and their work. The writers of the book, *Success Built to Last*, suggest that this attitude is born in us while we are in the process of determining the core values that will govern our lives. They write, on another level, that organizations that seek to survive and grow are led in a study that is completed when they have put the core values of their enterprise or business on paper and commit to following them. In these sessions, they seek to come up with the list of values that they think they need to consider and follow if they are going to complete a successful assignment successfully.

In a predecessor book, *Built to Last*, these authors had learned that you do not or cannot create core ideologies: you discover them. They "are not derived by looking to the external environment: you get at it (them) by looking inside." You do not ask what core values should we hold. You ask instead, "What core values do we actually hold?"

The intimation is, you learn what your core values are by looking back, not by looking ahead. They are not goals; they are attitudes that exist while we are in the process of doing. They literally shout out at us while we are engaged in living, and we don't have the chance to see what they are until we reflect on what we have done. Then we see what caused us to do what we have done, and those causes are the core values with which we are living. They are, of course, open to change.

The authors use, as an illustration, the situation of former President Jimmy Carter. They reflect, "After a crushing defeat, he created his new definition of success that, when you meet him, you're certain is much more meaningful to him than any that came before. He found a much better job—one that he's done for more than a quarter century and will do for the rest of his life." The values that governed his life changed after he discovered what he wanted to be.

The authors of *Success* finally decided that "what helps successful people stay successful is their stubbornness about sticking with their own journey based on their own values, not on a magic path following precisely by everyone else. There is no more personal decision than to discover what meaning means to you. And only you can make that choice."

During our later years, we have the chance to think back upon the decisions we have made and the paths we have traveled in our lives to see what is important to us. Then as we contemplate the years to come, we can decide if we are satisfied with what we have done and how we have done it, or—if we have been moving in another and wrong direction—they we can decide if a change in direction needs to be made.

Sixty-Six

What Will the Second Half of Our Lives Be About?

I fell in love with the epilogue in Denis Waitley's writing, *Empires of The Mind*. It was a great ending for his book, though I think it would also have made a great beginning. Read on with me: "One of the greatest lessons I've learned"—writes Waitley—"in life is that success is neither the destination nor the journey, but a way of traveling. Destinations and journeys inevitably involve arrivals and endings."

"I've always felt"—again Waitley—"that the word *retired* was misspelled. The word should be *retried* or maybe *reinspired*. A commencement ceremony after one career or major achievement should bring with it the anticipation of another peak experience ahead, challenging and enriching our bodies, minds, and souls in new creative pursuits."

Waitley concludes:

> "I like the idea of life being an endless range of mountains with peaks and valleys, inclines and descents, and always more peaks ahead to climb."

> "Life is not something to step back from and admire when completed. It is an ongoing process, laying foundations, forming, erecting, bonding, changing, detailing, refining, and renovating."

> "Life calls for the cathedral perspective. It calls for us to gain hindsight from all that went before. It calls for us to live in the present, longing for neither yesterday nor tomorrow, but rather, facing what today offers boldly, optimistically and flexibly."

> "Life, like a cathedral, is not so much to be admired for its external appearance and majesty, although those are attractive and noteworthy. Life, like a cathedral, is more meaningful because of what goes on in the sanctity within."

And then this last line:

> "Hasten not to build your cathedrals or conquer your empires. Seek patiently and persistently to discover them by looking inward."

There is a whole lot of wisdom in those words! Think about it. We build the first part of our lives brick by brick with materials which we can see and experience, even as others can see and experience it and them. We start our growing-up years at home and in our neighborhood, learning from our parents and playmates. We graduate to elementary, junior, and senior high school. We move on to learn more in our college years and, if we are lucky, through some post-graduate experiences. Then we hit the real world. Forty or so years later, we lay all of that experience aside with, as Waitley suggests, "a commencement event that prepares us for another experience." We then seek to be reinspired!

The problem is that the second half of life, following our retirement ceremony, is harder to define and create. There are no road maps for that part of our lives. We are on our own with our suitcase of experience, left to wonder, "Where do I go from here?"

Then comes his final sentence, and read it well:

> "Hasten not to build your cathedrals or conquer your empires. Seek patiently and persistently to discover them by looking inward."

It will take a real effort to decide what next to build or where else to go. But it will be time well spent if we take those days, months, or even years to plot out our tomorrow years. So open the door and walk down the aisle of the cathedral you want to build with your new life, and enjoy your second or third life!

Sixty-Seven

We Need to Let Our Lives Speak to Us!

What on earth am I to do with the rest of my life? Let me share some words, in answer to this question, from a devotional commentary in *The 2006 Upper Room Disciplines: A Book of Daily Devotions*. Heidi Schlumpf writes, "How do we know the task to which we are being called?" There is certainly not an easy and apparent answer to such a question. We might yearn for a distinct voice, for a clear sign for a transparent word that would answer such a question for us. However, let us remember that even for the Hebrew prophet called Isaiah, the call did not come that way. God did not speak directly to him. Instead, Isaiah overhears God speaking to someone else, lamenting to the heavenly court about who might be sent on God's behalf to accomplish a particular task that was at hand. The prophet, cleansed and purified, however, responded with a resounding, "Here I am. Send me!" Perhaps we need to possess a readiness to overhear our call no matter how it comes and be ready to respond to it.

The genius is in being open enough and ready and willing to listen to what life might have to say to us. Too often we find ourselves overwhelmed by our own intended ideas, by our busyness, and by our desire to accomplish some great thing; in the process, we miss hearing the still small voice that life might be using to speak to us.

I have made reference to Denis Waitley's words about the second half of life as being a time to be reinspired; to be ready to retry some of the things, opportunities, or ideas that we discarded early on in our lives while we were in the process of seeking to accomplish what we assumed were to be our life's intended goals. At that time in our life, we were intent on making our parents and ourselves proud!

During the second half of our lives—that is, after we have completed the intentions that guided us through the initial years of our lives while we were being led by the continuing question, "What do you want to be when you grow up?"—we have the opportunity to rethink the direction of our anticipations. Now we have the chance to listen, for the first time perhaps, to those voices with and around us that may suggest some other avenue of adventure that might satisfy us for the remainder of our lives.

The opportunities are certainly there. Some new venture, some new enterprise, or some new dream or aspiration. The problem is in seeing it with one's own eyes, or hearing it with one's own mind or ear.

Tired? Ready to relax? But not ready to lie down? Is that what Waitley was writing about; what Ms. Schlumpf had in mind in her devotional moment? And again, how is life going to speak to us? Not, perhaps, in some direct conversation, but quietly, subconsciously, almost inaudibly. The responsibility is ours. We have to do the listening! We have to be waiting to hear about our next assignment! Ours! Mine! Those are the objects of life's intended directions. We have to determine how to reach that point in our second life when we are able to listen and to hear. What was the biblical word? "Speak, Lord, for thy servant is listening." Maybe!

Sixty-Eight

We Need to Find the Time to Start Our Lives over Again!

In his novel *Point of No Return*, John Marquand speaks of a man who, after years of apple-polishing and bucking for promotion and dedicating all his energies to a single goal, finally attained it and becomes vice president of the fancy but little New York Bank where he works. It is at that particular moment in time that he realizes that what he has accomplished was not what he really wanted after all; the prize that he had spent his life trying to win suddenly turns to ashes in his hands. His promotion assures him and his family all the security and standing that he has sought, but Marquand leaves you with the feeling that maybe the best way Charlie Gray could have supported his family would have been by giving his life to the kind of work where he could have expressed and fulfilled himself in such a way as to become, in himself as a person, the kind of person they really needed.

At some point in time, perhaps we discover that we have accomplished what we thought we wanted to accomplish only to find out that in it we have no final sense of fulfillment. Then Marquand reminds us, as Frederick Buechner suggests, "Surely Marquand was right when he writes that for each one of us, there comes a point of no return, a point beyond which we no longer have life enough left to go back and start all over again." But when does one arrive at *that moment* in time? I suspect that it is different for each and every one of us. Consequently, we need to be on the lookout for that crossroads in our lives. We might pass by it without knowing it, and in that fleeting moment, our lives will be found for the final finish.

If I found myself having accomplished what I believe to be the fulfillment of my life's dream, realizing that I had climbed a ladder set against the wrong wall, the question becomes, "How do I move the ladder to a wall where I can start climbing again toward the goal that *maybe* life has set before me?" Another question then raises its hoary head: "How much time do I need to best what I thought to be my life's work?"

Certainly, as long as we have enough breath, we can start over: begin a new life with new goals and aspirations. Age is not necessarily a burden. The need is to reflect on one's past to see if there has been a time when one would like to have started over but knew the responsibilities of one's family obligations made it impossible to visit the land of beginning again.

However, as one approaches the beginning of life number 2, following retirement—well, maybe the chance is there to start over again? It just demands some serous reflection and the tug of a life not completely satisfied to start one off in a new direction. Each day offers us the possibility of a new beginning, even if that new beginning is long in coming or if there are a number of new beginnings. One's possible new life is only hindered by one's lack of optimism and sense of desire.

Where do I want to go? What will it take to get me to the next starting block? What plans will I need to make as I survey the present and the future?

Sixty-Nine

We Need to Think about Yesterday Today!

I looked in the mirror this morning, and the person I saw today was the same one that I think I saw yesterday; it was not. I am not the same person I was yesterday. Isn't that what they say about our bodies? Cells live and cells die to be replaced by new cells. Our whole body is in a constant state of change and redevelopment. I am not the same person I was yesterday, and that, in more ways than one.

M. Scott Peck suggests that we ought to be smarter than our parents: that we cannot assume that all that they taught us is right today; rather, it is always open to investigation. His words, "There is no such thing as a good hand-me-down religion. To be vital, to be the best of which we are capable, our religion must be a wholly personal one, forged entirely through the fire of our questioning and doubting in the crucible of our own experience of reality." Then these words, "The path to 'holiness' lies through questioning everything." Let me extend his words: "The path to 'wholeness' lies through questioning everything." I think it was the Greek philosopher Socrates who offered up this observation: "The unexamined life is not worth living."

Does this suggest to you, as it does to me, that we ought to be regularly reinvestigating what we think and pondering what we are doing before we move on to another stage in our living? I have been reading a book that has challenged the way I think about one thing and another. I can understand what the author is trying to say, but

I am completely at odds with his conclusions. The point is that my reading of his words has caused me to rethink what I believe. Not what I believe in, but what I believe!

Are we not wiser ourselves than we were yesterday? If that is true, and it probably is, then we should be regularly rethinking what we are doing and where we are going, particularly at that time in our lives when we have no boundaries to hold us in and no responsibilities to hold us back—meaning today!

The second part of our living, someone has called it life number 2, there is so much freedom in it, yet we don't seem to realize that we can use that freedom so much differently than we did in life number 1. Reading, listening, watching—they add to our knowledge, and if questioning is an option, then we need to focus all that we are today on what we are doing today so that tomorrow we can perhaps do things differently and move on in a new, more interesting and challenging direction.

I have limited responsibilities today. My family is raised. My day job is now a thing of the past, and my financial resources are not dependent on my day-to-day living. Wow! What freedom! Now all I have to do is to determine what I want to do with the rest of my life; on my life today, and then tomorrow.

In a real sense, my life today has nothing to do with yesterday because I am not the same person. Today I have more resources mentally; fiscally; and, to a degree, physically than I had when I began life number 1! If time allows, I have the opportunity to begin a whole new life!

History tells us that our forefathers, upon their arrival in the new world, began their journey on Ellis Island. After their long journey, now they stood ready to take advantage of the great promise that awaited them. A new world! A new way of life! Look around you? See what their hands have wrought! Think about what *you* could do if you put your mind to it!

To paraphrase M. Scott Peck, "to be vital, to be the best of which I am capable, my life must be wholly personal, one forged through the fire of our questioning and doubting in the crucible of my own experience of reality." So today, at that moment when I shut down my computer, I have the chance to reassess where I am, and in the light of what I think I ought to be doing, I can begin to walk in a new direction to accept the opportunities of a new journey. Wow! The possibilities are endless. They just have to be within the realm of reality, as far as my circumstances and situation and resources are concerned.

"I'm thinking! I'm thinking!" (Think, Jack Benny!)

SEVENTY

Is the World Waiting for Your Second Coming-Out Party?

I ran into a rather interesting observation the other day. It came from the pen of Theodore Roosevelt who had this thought to offer: "Far and away, the best prize that life offers is the chance to work hard at work worth doing." The hope is that each and every one of us chooses a vocation that allows us to satisfy this dream. Some of us will find ourselves satisfied by several vocational adventures, maybe even more in this day and age when job transition seems to be in vogue.

When it comes to the second half of life however, during those years we spend following the completion of our so-called life work, that is another tale altogether. What do we do with all the energy and resources that we bring to the table once we have begun to receive a monthly check from the Social Security Administration? The question that arises is, "At this stage in our lives, what kind of work or labor do we think is worth doing? How do we want to invest the special days that our industry, in the first half of life, is now able to underwrite?"

People today are perpetual volunteers, and we could not do without them and the jobs that they accomplish. We see many such individuals in the hospitals that we visit at the reception desk, in the gift shop, pushing book carts in the hall, delivering mail or the daily paper. Others of us find our satisfaction in serving on one community board or another, using the time we have been given to serve the community in which we live. Some of us tutor in the local school district. Others of us continue in our former vocation, though now we do the job for free or for a fraction of what we might have earned or charged earlier.

Some of us, however, will find ourselves unsatisfied by each and every one of these extracurricular avocations. Some of us need more substance in our lives.

I remember reading of Crawford Greenawalt, the CEO—I think it was—of the Dupont Corporation. Early in his life, he became enamored with butterflies. He determined to give one hour every day of his life to the study of those beautiful creatures of creation that we see flying from here to there in the summer sky. Later in life, he was recognized for the knowledge he had accumulated on the subject over the years. He became a source of information for others who had a similar interest. He made it in the business world, in *his* world, but he never tired of his hobby; and the world was the beneficiary of his personal discipline.

How about making some subject or area of expertise your life adventure? Yes, you might have to make a late start, say like today; but in any event, in what area of interest and concern might you now invest the remaining years of your life? Think about all the experience and/or information that you have accumulated over the years? What kind of impact can you make upon the worlds in which you now live with the background that you bring to today's table? What might you have to do to bring yesterday's experience into today's world in a fresh new way? What kind of difference might you make in the place where you live, work, and play today!

Now you have the time. Think about it, and with the help of your local library or your local university or through the Elderhostel movement, make yourself fluent in your special area of interest and reach out to the world around you. It may turn out to be a very personal adventure, one known only to yourself, and all you will get out of it is a sense of self-satisfaction. On the other hand, the world might be waiting for you to have a second coming-out party.

I don't know what interests you might have, and maybe right now, you don't either; *but* the world can be yours when all you have is time and energy to invest! Wow! That idea excites me. I hope that it excites you!

Seventy-One

We All Have but One Life to Live! Use It Well!

I read a while ago of the passing of Clifford Goertz. He was reputed to be the leading cultural anthropologist of his era. Goertz is said to have observed that we all start out with the possibility of living a thousand different lives, but we end up living only one. Late in his life, he also noted "a lot of people don't quite know where they are going…but I don't even know, for certain, where I have been." He did conclude, however, that along with many others in the postwar (World War II) era, he had lived a charmed life in a charmed time. Goertz said he doubted whether such an opportune time in history would ever come again.

Isn't that the hope of all of us, to live a "charmed life in a charmed time"? Goertz was led into his professional life by an individual whom he thought of as a mentor. The helper suggested, near the end of the World War, that he apply to the avant-garde Antioch College in Yellow Springs, Ohio. He did, and that move, with the help of the G.I. Bill, propelled him into a distinguished academic career.

Avenues of possibility are ever open to all of us. We read of them. We hear about them. We are directed to them by individuals whom we know in ways beyond our imagining. And if we are fortunate enough to find our way, then we will have the life that we have always been looking for. The point is, it takes some work, some thought, some real effort; and a willingness to keep our eyes and ears open.

I don't know if I can say that I have lived a "charmed life," or that the times in which I have lived have been "charmed times" though I grew up in much the same world as Professor Goertz. In reflection, I know that I missed a couple of turns in the road, made some rather stupid decisions, and passed by some wonderful opportunities and times because I either was too busy to see them and capitalize on them, or was too lazy to move in their direction.

I guess what I am thinking is that those lifetime possibilities are forever before us. Until we take our last breath, we stand close to a road or path or a trail that could lead us into a time that will be a blessing for each one of us. Maybe not a charmed life, but certainly a charmed time in the midst of one's life—and what better time for that than in one's senior or later years?

Oh, we can't move as fast as we might like, and there are some journeys that are too long or involved to be completed now within the length of our lives on this planet; but there are some possibilities out there right in front of our eyes, waiting to be seen and hoping to be found! What are they as far as I or you are concerned? Think now! Rack your memory bank? Some new or some old, anticipated desire or dream, still unfulfilled, presently forgotten? If I find one that appeals to me, maybe I ought to set down a timeline that will help me to accomplish its fulfillment. And even if I don't arrive at my destination, I will at least leave this life moving in the right direction.

Goertz said that "we start out with the possibility of living a thousand different lives, but we end up living only one." Frankly, I am not so sure he was right. I believe that today, we can all live more than one life in our lifetime, and I am going to try my best at doing it.

Seventy-Two

Here's a New Way of Thinking About Life in the Present Tense!

I saw an advertisement in the morning newspaper. It's lead sentence reported: "Boomers are reinventing retirement." Now it was a marketing point for a financial company, and it had to do with one's investment portfolio. However, it seemed to me that it was also saying something else that all of us, in the midst of our living these days, needs to think about.

Retirement is being reinvented! It used to be an age, sixty-five years of age for the average worker; and even for military personnel and educational workers who thought of twenty or thirty years as a retirement objective, it spoke of retirement. People planned for that day and offered a sigh of relief when it arrived.

Today, however, we are told that seventy-two is the new sixty-five, and maybe sixty-five is the new fifty. The point is, people are not ready to sit down and rock today when they reach the age of sixty-five. Rather, they are ready to move on in a new direction to find new avenues of employment or an additional means of fulfillment when they reach that magic age. And rightly so. Our energies are just recuperating; our internal engines are just revving up now at that "old-time" retirement age.

So as we have been suggesting, one has to begin planning for that time, whether it comes earlier or later than sixty-five. What am I going to do then or now? Many of us will not even pause on our journey. We are ready and willing to work until we fall down from exhaustion or worse. Our desk chair will not be getting cold for quite a while. We don't know how to slow down. We don't want to slow down, so we just keep going, fueled by some internal energizer bunny.

It is the same song, only a new verse, to what has been written on the previous pages. Keep going! Keep on going! Keep thinking! Keep on thinking! Rest and then move on and continue your adventure, even if it is in a new direction. As Winston Churchill told a graduating class in Great Britain, "Never give up! Never give up! Never give up!" And we won't. Even if we have some sort of medical problem.

Perhaps we have lost some of our energy or our mobility. I read recently about one of the politicians whose name is familiar to many of us. He suggested that many of his peers, with similar or dissimilar experiences, have a lot to offer to the world around them. He said that they ought to get together and talk about the problems that face their worlds with the thought that the results of those conversations would have some significant impact on the problems being faced by people who are much younger who don't have the experience of those who are older.

This is why biographies and autobiographies and reflective writings by so many gifted people are so much in demand. We don't want to hear about their prejudices and their gripes. We do, however, want to hear some of their observations. We want to know what they think because they have already been where we are and where we are going, and their ideas might save us from making the same mistakes that they made or that we might make.

We need to spend some time recouping our wisdom, sharing it with others not as the unvarnished truth but as an idea that others might use to sandpaper their ideas and aspirations. It is not so much that boomers are reinventing retirement; it is that they are reinventing life, and maybe we can help them…

Seventy-Three

How to Write a Happy Ending to the Story of Your Life!

I read recently of the accomplishments of a psychiatrist by the name of Dr. George Vaillant. He embarked on a rather ambitious long-term study of young men from different backgrounds. He hoped to identify traits in the young men, in their teens and twenties, that would predict successful careers and home lives when they were in their forties, and contented old age when they were older.

Writing in the final volume of his study report entitled, *Aging Well*, Vaillant reports that he was pleased to learn that for many people, "Old age did not have to be a time of loss, regret, and playing out the string. Rather, just as the final innings of a baseball game are often more exciting than the earlier ones, just as more typically happens in the last twenty minutes of a movie than in the first twenty, just as many a good book comes together and begins to make sense in the last few chapters, so a person's last years, if done right, can be, in the words of Robert Browning, 'The last of life for which the first was made.'"

He identified two primary keys to have contentment late in life. The first was to have a growing circle of friendships. He would urge us to make a deliberate effort to cultivate new friendships as old friends move out of our lives due to death or relocation. He suggested that we should go as far as to take a personal social inventory of our lives every six to twelve months, asking ourselves, "Have I made a new friend recently?"

The second key is to be found, he writes, in nurturing our ability to forgive slights and injuries. We ought to spend as much or more time looking forward to our future as we do contemplating our past. We ought to take the effort to look back with gratitude more than with regret and with more fondness than with bitterness. Writing in his book, *The Progress Paradox*, Gregg Easterbrook made a similar point. "People are happy if they are optimistic, grateful, and forgiving. If we think only about our disappointments and unsatisfied wants, we may be prone to unhappiness. If, on the other hand, we are aware of our disappointments but at the same time are thankful for the good, then contentment comes more easily."

In Vaillant's words, "People who make lemonade out of lemons fare better (in old age) than people who turn molehills into mountains." Another, Thomas Moore writes, "I have made many mistakes and done a lot of foolish things, and when I look back at the person I was, I feel affection for him."

Vaillant found that people who were unhappy in their late years were suffering not from a lack of material things but from a lack of love, companionship, and optimism. In one of his key findings, he writes, "It is not the bad things that happened to us that doom us, but the good people who happened to us at any age that facilitate an enjoyable old age."

Score one for the suggestion that we ought to spend more time drinking coffee in a coffee shop than sitting at our family table. I am a loner who is prone to sit at the kitchen table. Well, even though coffee is overpriced down at the corner restaurant, I think I will give the bar stool at the counter a try to see who I can meet. Life is longer than we might expect, and a lonely life is not what was intended for most of us. I need to be engaged in writing a happy ending to my life! How about you?

SEVENTY-FOUR

There Is Importance to be Found in the Process of "Becoming."

I like this thought: "True success consists not in becoming the person you dreamed of being when you were young, but in becoming the person you were meant to be; the person you are capable of being when you are your best."

Interestingly enough, it is a job that one can accomplish only later in life, after the activities and shouting have died down and we are left to ourselves to ponder where we are and how we got there. It is in those moments that we have the opportunity to wonder, perhaps out loud, "Is or was that all there is?" or "Is there or was there to be *more*"?

We miss so much during our earning years! We are so busy going from here to there that we don't have time to stop and face the needs around us, or the one's within us: "To smell," as someone has suggested, "the roses." We are up early in the morning, spend our days moving in one forward direction or another or perhaps in a backward direction, and we then fall exhausted into bed in the evening and are hardly ready, the next morning, to do it all over again. But we have to, and so we do!

The later years can afford us the opportunity to lie in bed or sit on the couch and vegetate, and we have earned the right to do that; and some of us are. But finally, if we have an ounce of industry in us, we will say, as someone did to me so many years ago, "I have planted as many tulips as I want to."

Another: a successful business type who was soon to leave for his winter home in Carefree, Arizona, "You can only play so much golf!" Some, I must quickly add, never get enough of that!

But many of us do, and I am one of them. We want to be more productive! Maybe it means standing in the lobby of a store and welcoming people who come to shop. Just smiling and passing out some positive reinforcement. For others, it may mean a new career, or the exploring of some new interests through organizations such as Elderhostel. Who knows? What is important is for us to take the time to reconsider our dreams. Harold Kushner remarks, "The worth of a person's soul is not measured by the size of his or her bank account or the volume of the applause a person evokes, but by one's humanity, by one's compassion, even by the courage to keep on dreaming amid the broken pieces of earlier dreams."

Professor Philip Simmons, a gifted teacher debilitated by ALS at an early age, recalls vacationing with his family in New Hampshire one summer and offering to remove some large stones from the dirt that led up to their cabin. His father told him to leave the stones in place. "Without them, the dirt road would turn to mud when the rain came. We need a hard road," his father told him, "not a smooth one." And so we do, and the road will never end this side of heaven's gate.

Who am I? What have I become? What potential do I still have within me? I need to pick up the pieces of my life, as they are scattered around me, and move on in a forward direction! Are you with me?

Seventy-Five

How to Overcome Life's Disappointments!

I was truly intrigued by Rabbi Harold Kushner's writing, *Overcoming Life's Disappointments*. It is a good read. He opens a chapter, bearing the above title, with these words: "What does a person do with all the dreams that don't come true—dreams of emerging talents, dreams of career, dreams of wealth and recognition, dreams of marriage and family?" Then on another page, he adds this question, "How do you find the will to go on when you realize that the life you are living is not the one you have been looking forward to?"

Earlier in his book, he addressed the problems that Israelite leader Moses encountered when, in frustration, he hurled to the ground the two pieces of stone that bore the famed Ten Commandments that he had brought down from the mountaintop. Kushner suggests that after he had ascended the Sinai peak for the second time and descended with two new pieces of stone bearing the Decalogue, Moses cleaned up the pieces of the original tablets and put them in the Ark along *with* the set he had received on his second trip.

> "For Moses, the words on the first set of tablets, the ones carved by God, were demands that turned out to be too much for the people. The words on the second set, a joint effort of God and devoted humans, were a vision, a summons

to be more than we are, and as such, they endure to this day."

Did he answer his question with this imaginary act on the part of the Hebrew leader? Yes, we all had hopes and dreams in our early years. "I want to be a fireman, or a doctor, or a teacher, or an explorer, or…but I ended up working in a factory, being an accountant, a waste collector." So?

In our dreams, we can remember our aspirations, hopefully with a smile; and in the midst of the remains of those dreams, we can fashion a new life and be the best that we can be at it. The pieces in the Ark were a reminder to Moses of God's intentions for his people; the second set of stones made him aware of what he could do. What we can do and what we want to do are the grounds on which two distinct roads are to be built. The one leads to nowhere, the other leads to somewhere: the place where we are.

There is nothing wrong with aspirations, but our dreams have to be conditioned by reality; and when reality sets in, we need to use it to fashion a new set of dreams. We can handle the dreams that don't come true because one day we will see them only as dreams. We can adapt to the life we are living because, in our maturity, we will see it as the result of our gifts, our abilities, and our heritage. We can find comfort, vision, and drive in such a reality. Perhaps they are God's dream for us come true!

SEVENTY-SIX

The Importance of Summing Up Your Life!

We are probably the last people who really knew them. I mean your kids' parents, or your grandchildren's grand- and great-grandparents. The thought that follows came to me after reading several paragraphs in Frederick Buechner's writing, *Listening to Your Life*.

He writes: "It is so easy to sum up other people's lives...and necessary too, of course, especially our parents' lives. It is a way of reducing their giant figures to a size we can manage. I suppose, a way of getting even, maybe; of getting on; of saying goodbye! The day will come when somebody will try to sum you up the same way and also me. 'Tell me about old Buechner then. What was he really like? What made him tick? How did his story go? Well, you see, this happened and then that happened, and then that; and that is why he became thus and so, and why when all is said and done, it is not so hard to understand why things turned out for him as they finally did.'" He writes more, but you get the drift.

The thought before me is, my parents and grandparents: they are a part of my kids' and grandkids' lives, and whether they care or not, we have the responsibility of passing on some of their heritage to the later generations. They may not care, and that is fine; but *we have the responsibility to pass it one*!

Several years ago, my daughter gave me a book. It was entitled *Grandpa!* Tell me you promptly put it away and lost it, but Buechner's words suddenly brought me up short. My kids and grandkids don't know the whole of it. Oh, there are things that I would never tell them that I never told anyone; only God knows about them, and that is just fine. But the book was/is filled with the opportunity to write down my history for what it is worth.

Since my parents saw my children only several times a year—and those weren't always good meetings—they are a distant blessing; and whether we realize it or not, their lives and their decisions have had a tremendous impact on who I am and, subsequently, on who my children are.

So off to the store I am going to buy the book so that I can pass on my memories to those whom I love. I think to myself, *Who cares?*, and maybe nobody does; but history is something of importance to all of us, and I need to write down a bit more.

The challenge is there for all of us. For some of us, it will be easier than for others. Some of us will create a pictorial history. Sadly, as I think about it now, we didn't take a whole lot of pictures. So the challenge is there for all of us. Grandpa! Grandma! Tell me your story! Write down some history!

SEVENTY-SEVEN

We Need to Remember the Gifts That We Have Received When Life Gets Us Down!

I remember reading the story of a man who was about to retire. During his company party, a man whom he hardly knew approached him to tell him how much he had appreciated his leadership and how much he would miss him. He said, "I decided not to go in with the others in purchasing a gift. I wanted to give you something myself. I didn't know, however, what that ought to be. Finally, I decided upon this." He pulled something out of his pocket. When he opened his fingers, which were hiding it, the gift was revealed. It was his pocketknife. Worn from decades of going everywhere with him, indispensable to a man who was very self-sufficient: here was a gift that could be used to cut up an apple, shorten a rope, or a piece of string. It could be used to fix things.

"If someone would have asked me," the retiring man said, "to list five hundred things you might vaguely hope to possess one day, I would never have thought of a gift like that. I would never have said, 'Hey, a pocketknife is what I want.' But here was this invaluable gift being placed in my hand."

Then the giver offered these words of presentation, "Carry this around with you in your pocket. Then someday, when you're having a bad day, feel it down in there and remember that someone loves you."

He knew that he had to attach some words to his gift. "When you are having a bad day, feel it down in there, and remember that someone loves you." It's true, is it not, that we are not always sure what to make of the stuff that comes our way? However, when we meet whatever it is, how easy it is to confront it when we have words like this in our possession: "Remember, when you are having a bad day, feel it down in there, and remember that somebody loves you."

My shelves are filled, so it seems, with small, little underappreciated gifts given to me by one person or another over the years: items from friends with whom I have lived and worked, cards from my children and grandchildren, and from my spouse. It is those special treasures that I can turn to when life seems to be getting me down. I just swivel my desk chair around and look at those shelves and those tokens of appreciation and love, and suddenly all is right in my world.

What is on your shelf? What have you accumulated over the years that you can use to help you combat any of the difficulties that come your way? Poor health, discouragement, a sense of lostness? "A pocketknife! A word of compassion and care: 'Carry that around with you in your pocket. Then someday, when you are having a bad day, feel it down in there and remember that somebody loves you.'"

Let me tell you about some of the things that I have on my shelf. Better yet, think about it: what do you have on your shelves that you can count on when life seems to be getting you down?

SEVENTY-EIGHT

We Need to Look at Life from Every Direction.

I chanced upon this story the other day. Alexander Schmemann, the late priest who led a reform in Russian orthodoxy, tells of a time when he was travelling on the subway in Paris, France, with his fiance. At one stop, an old and ugly woman dressed in the uniform of the Salvation Army got on and found a seat nearby. The two lovers whispered to each other in Russian about how repulsive she looked. A few stops later, the woman stood to exit. As she passed them, she said in perfect Russian, "I wasn't always ugly!" Schmemann would later tell his students, "That woman was an angel of God." She opened his eyes, searing his vision in a way he would never forget.

The story awakened me to a fact of my age and time in life. Those of us who are older are, too often, one-dimensional in our thinking. We see action, events, and situations from a one-dimensional point of view. More often than not, that point of view is selfish; very self-centered. Older people are described as being selfish and wanting everything for nothing. It is almost as if we believe the world owes us something. Now maybe it does owe many of my generation something, but there are only a few individuals who fall into that category.

Bearing that in mind and with this story fresh on my mind, it reminded me of the fact that as I grow older, I need to become more multidimensional in my approach to life. I need to stand back in almost every situation in which I find myself and consider the whole of it before I dive in with some complaint or criticism. Earlier on, I suggested that people my age need to listen more and talk less.

Schmemann's experience ought to remind us that, again, too often we see things only from our immediate point of view. We need to follow the old saying, "Before you criticize an Indian, you need to walk away in his moccasins."

We need to learn that the world *does not* owe us a living and that all we can see is not enough. I can't get that comment out of my mind: "I wasn't always ugly!" I would suggest that she was saying to her critics that life had been hard on her, and *that* hardness had not been all her fault. How many times had she been at the wrong place at the wrong time? I suspect that I have had some bad moments in my life when I have been in much the same situation. I wasn't ready for an event or a problem, and my poor response to it played a significant role in my development, negatively speaking. We can grow ourselves ugly if we are not careful.

The challenge is to try to see life from a variety of perspectives to root out the background of a person or a situation before we wade in with some comment that needs to be thought through before it is voiced publicly. I have nothing but time, so I ought to use it more wisely.

My generation has so much to share with the world. We have been there and done that! We need to carefully examine each word before we voice it and each criticism before we make it. The world will be a better place when more of us do that. "I wasn't always ugly"? One wonders, what was her former life like? And now this: Who around me needs some positive input before I make some negative comment?

SEVENTY-NINE

The Search for Meaning is a Continuing Journey!

In their book *Success Built to Last*, the authors are speaking to the general theme, "Creating a life that matters!" They touch upon a nerve, at least in my life, when they offer up this thought, "Too many people, at some point in their lives, set goals and go on to achieve them, often brilliantly, only to find that they are mysteriously disappointed, empty, and unhappy. Could this be why, despite acquiring luxuries undreamed of even a few decades ago, that there is a rising epidemic of clinical depression and suicide among the wealthiest citizens in America, China, and other rapidly growing economies?"

> "How is it possible to achieve the very definition of success and yet find happiness so fleeting? Builders (enduringly successful people) say it's a simple matter of being cheated by the absence of knowing what really matters to you in your life not just for today but for today and the long term."

It's the question of looking back over one's formative years, deciding what was important back there and then determining whether or not, during the course of the following years, one kept faith with that vision or somehow, over the course of those years, got so engrossed in doing a particular job or accomplishing some extraneous vision that they lost sight of what they had hoped their lives would be all about.

Once we receive "our gold watch for service and a job well-done," is it not important that, in some reflective moments, we revisit our lives to make sure that we accomplished what we set out to do? If we have, well and good, and we can continue our journey on the path we are walking. We can kick off our shoes, put up our feet, and relax!

On the other hand, it is possible that upon reflection, we will realize that somewhere during our life's journey we lost our way; and contrary to what other people might choose to believe, we didn't arrive at that place in life that we had been planning to go.

Now as we stand at the beginning of life number 2, the possibility exists for us to start over in a new way: to seek to satisfy the dream or aspiration that we, all at once, realize we did not satisfy. The acts of suicide or self-destruction that the authors mentioned—the rising epidemic of clinical depressions among the successful—is it not possible for us to avoid those dismal and discouraging moments by spending some of our time in honest self-examination, admitting to ourselves that though we were successful in the ways of the world and in the eyes of our peers, that we, ourselves, don't yet feel the sense of satisfaction that we want to feel? Maybe it is time for us to point our lives in a new direction.

Is it ever too late to begin again? I don't think so. It is just a matter of rethinking our priorities and expending the later energetic years of our lives reviewing, rethinking, and then recommitting ourselves to that first goal or vision. It is not a matter of ending it all in frustration. Rather, today offers us the opportunity to begin to walk in the direction we had originally planned to go sometime in the now-distant past.

Happy thinking! Happy hunting! Enjoy the rest of your life!

Eighty

We Are Our Secrets!

When I was a young person, growing up, I remember that many of the girls that I knew kept diaries. Little books with a lock to keep them private. Now I know that the locks were rather flimsy, easily broken, I am sure; but when the lock was broken, the writer immediately knew that someone had invaded their privacy. However, the purpose of the diary remained the same. The writer wrote down their secret thoughts sometime during the day. My granddaughter told me the other day that she had a diary! Now she is only learning to write, but she tells me that she writes things down; and when one might happen to read them and they can't because she keeps the book "locked," they would be able to tell what she was thinking. I am sure that it would be a priceless experience because she is a very interesting little girl.

Today, adults do journaling. I guess that is a more sophisticated kind of diary writing. In any event, I kept a journal for a number of years. Then, at intervals, I removed the writings from the loose-leaf notebook in which they had been placed and destroyed them. My problem is, being a very private person, I did not want someone else to know what I was thinking.

Then I came across, again, the wonderful writing of Dag Hammarsjold, the former secretary general of the United Nations, which he or someone else entitled, "Markings." Published after his death, it is a book filled up with wonderful thoughts and remembrances of what he thought each night as he came home from the office and wrote his reflections down on paper. I have read it a number of times.

Then these words of Frederick Buechner confronted me, "To keep track of these lives we live is not just a means of enriching our understanding and possibly improving our sermons (Buechner is a Presbyterian minister), but a truly sacred work. In these pages, I tell about my parents, my children, and myself because that is one way of keeping track, and because I believe that it is not only more honest but also vastly more interesting than to pretend that I have no such secrets to tell. 'I not only have secrets. I am my secrets.' And you are your secrets. Our secrets are human secrets, and our trusting each other enough to share them with each other has much to do with the secret of what it is to be human."

Now, frankly, I still do not feel free enough to write down my thoughts for others to read, sometime, somewhere, but I do think it is a good idea. I think I might start to write a journal again, and if I die in the process, before I go through the ritual of shredding my thoughts, someone might catch a glimpse of what I am thinking at this time in my life. They might be surprised! They might be horrified! Satisfied that they knew me, like they thought they knew me. But that is only an outside possibility because I will probably, periodically, destroy the writings.

But for you, maybe it is a good idea. Maybe you are freer within your skin that I am.

Buechner said, "I not only have secrets. I am my secrets!" And what better information to pass on from one generation to another; statements about what we are, what we have done, and what we wanted to be! Happy writing!

Eighty-One

Life Is a Team Effort!

The following words came to my attention in a book that I have been reading: "Thinking big about how we can reach the entire world might overwhelm us. But we can simply start where we are. What we do today has an impact both now and in the years to come." These sentences include a challenge and a way to satisfy it!

I think of watching a relay race being run by a team of great sprinters. Each one of them is a world champion in their own right on any given day. The initial runner stretches out his legs and runs for all he is worth, while the second runner, in his place, waits enthusiastically to do the same thing. The third and fourth runners await their turns as well. Individually, each one of the sprinters can only maintain the expected pace for a prescribed distance, but together they can run the race that is set before them and finish it in record time.

In the later years of our lives, as we reflect on our life and our attainments, we soon realize that we did not accomplish all that we had intended to do. We did not set the world on fire as we anticipated we would do in our childhood dreams. We found that we got sidetracked. We soon understood that, many times, we were not adequate to the challenges that our individual lives and careers threw at us. Yes, we tried! We worked hard! We sweat and we strained, both figuratively and in reality. But we did not get the job done, and in the quiet, reflective moments of our retirement, we know what we did not do.

I think of one particular corporation led by one great leader after another. As each assumed the mantle of leadership, he changed the way that the organization did its business. Individually, they bought one new business or another and sold businesses that their predecessors had purchased. Each one of the men, in their turn, did what they thought was right at the moment. Now years later, as we look back at their achievements and accomplishments, we find that the corporation is much better than it was years ago when the first of these men assumed the mantle of leadership. Each man's abilities complimented the genius of his predecessor. Whether they realized it or not, at the time, they were all runners in a relay race!

All of us, no matter what our occupation or place in life, need to be team players. We need to prepare our job for the person who will follow us with the hope that they will succeed where we have failed because they have the attributes that were needed when they assumed the office: that they have the gifts that we did not have.

All of us, in the process we call life, need to be team players: participants in a relay race. We need to prepare the job we are doing or have done for our successor or successors. Always, we need to hold on to the hope that they will succeed where we have failed because they have the attributes that we needed when they assumed the office: gifts that we do not and did not have.

Even now, today, in the winding down years of our lives, we need to be involved in preparing the present and the future for those who will follow in our footsteps. We maintain our homes and our property for those who will live in them in the years to come. We involve ourselves in the activities and life of the communities in which we live, presuming to leave behind the foundation that others will build upon in the years to come.

We seek to bequeath to the members of our family a heritage that they can be proud of; memories that will encourage them to continue their lives in the tradition that their foremothers and forefathers have struggled to maintain. We need to remember that we cannot change the world by ourselves, but as a part of a team, we can do wonderful things in it and for it. We just have to be big enough to realize our limitations and champion the abilities of those who will follow us.

It is never too late for us to improve the present, utilize our gifts in its development, and prepare tomorrow for the coming of those who are coming along behind us. Right?

Eighty-Two

The Importance of Leaving a Legacy.

Are you on this planet to do something, or are you here for something to do? If you're on this planet to do something, then what is it? What difference will you make in the worlds where you live, work, or play before you go to sleep? What will be your legacy? Remember the question, "What will be your legacy?" And remember, it does not have a single, right, or even simple answer.

The aforementioned questions are posed by authors James Kouzes and Barry Poster in their book, *A Leader's Legacy*. Then they offer us this challenge: "By asking ourselves how we want to be remembered, we plant the seeds for living our lives as if we matter. By living each day as if we matter, we offer up our own unique legacy. By offering up our own unique legacy, we make the world a better place than we found it."

I want us to look at the aforementioned questions and the statement that follows on a personal level. How do we want the world to remember us? How do we want our family to remember us? Our legacy—what do we want it to be?

In the early days of our retirement—whether it be our first, our second, or our third—we have these questions to ask and answer. The only question I hope that we really have to answer is this one: How much more do we want to do? How much more energy do we want to expend helping others in our family, in our community, etc.?

What might be the consequences of another burst of energy on our part in one area of living or another in this world of ours?

After our first retirement party, perhaps we are most likely going to want to make some additional plans to accomplish some private goal or need. We have significant energy resources left, and we can reach out in many directions to involve ourselves in one project or another. As we get older, however, our energy level begins to deteriorate. Each passing year brings with it a certain amount of discomfort in one part of our body or another. I have found, however, that one particular passion or another can revive the enthusiasm that continues to inhabit our bodies. Such bursts of energy can propel us forward in one area or another for any number of years. Always, of course, we have the opportunity to just sit down and relax our lives away. Many of us, however, will not be content with that state of affairs. So we will keep looking for another opportunity or task in which to involve ourselves.

Maybe if we feel that we have not done enough, we ought to be involved in writing our own obituary. This will allow us the chance to chronicle our accomplishments and enable us to see what else we want to do: what else we can do to satisfy our questing spirit? This mock account of our lives will tell us what the world will remember about us. Maybe we ought to ask one family member and another to tackle writing our obituary along with us. The results of their labors will tell us how they will remember us.

Undoubtedly, they will have a whole other point of view. Merging these two viewpoints will go a long way toward giving us the opportunity to see ourselves as we really are and enable us, if we are so inclined, to make those personal changes we wish to make and ponder one new direction or another that we might still wish to travel.

In any event, the exercises mentioned above will go a long way toward allowing us to make plans that will help us to leave this world with a feeling of satisfaction. And if we do a good job, our family will already have an obituary ready when the time comes…

Eighty-Three

A Word about Yesterday's Challenge? Today's Quest?

I have been reading a book written by former Senator John Danforth of the Ralston Purina Danforths. Included early in his writing, *Faith and Politics*, Danforth has an autobiographical chapter in which he makes reference to a book written by his grandfather, entitled, *I Dare You!* It was written to promote his vision of the fourfold life. The four squares stood for the physical, the mental, the social, and the religious aspects of life. The third generation Danforth writes that "William Danforth coined a series of motivational slogans beginning with the words of his book title."

When I was a graduating senior in high school, I was given the I Dare You Award and was awarded a copy of the little red book that is mentioned above. I must confess that I never read the book, long ago discarded, probably by my parents when they broke up housekeeping and moved to the south. Hence, the three slogans rang like new when I read them:

I dare you to stand tall, think tall, smile tall, and live tall!
I dare you to be your own self at your very best ail of the time!
I dare you to aspire nobly, adventure daringly, serve humbly!

They are challenges that are worthy of reconsideration during the later years of our lives as well. Don't you agree? In other words, I can print them out and put them under glass on my desk and work at satisfying them, now today! In some ways, they are easier to do now with life three quarters gone. In other ways, they are perhaps more difficult since our time of adventure is much shorter.

Think about them yourself? "I dare you to stand tall, think tall, smile tall, and live tall." Physically, I have trouble standing tall. My back hurts. However, I can think tall, smile tall, and live tall. What those challenges mean for my life may be different than what they mean for your life, but I think I can do it. How about you?

I dare you to be your own self and be at your best all the time. I find it easier today to live within my own skin; though it is difficult, I admit, to sometimes be myself. As I get older, I gripe a lot more, and I do a lot less. How about you?

Finally, I dare you to aspire nobly, adventure daringly, and serve humbly! I wish I were more humble, and I hope I am becoming so every day. I do have some significant aspirations that I hope I can satisfy, because always, always, I am looking for a new direction for my life: for a new adventure to engage in during the latter years of my living.

How about you? Would you be willing to take these three challenges to heart and see what they can say to your life? They might change the direction of your living! They might change the worlds in which you live! They might change your life! Wow!

Eighty-Four

Reading Poses Some Life-Changing Possibilities!

I have a number of books on my to-read pile on the floor of my office that are about reading. One title suggests to me some new possibilities that are inherent in the books I have already read. It says that the contents of no book remains the same: that each time I read a book, because I am reading it at a different time and because I am a new person at that particular moment in time, that the book will have a new and special message for me.

I opened another book this morning and just read its introduction. It began with these words from the late Supreme Court Justice Oliver Wendell Holmes: "Man's mind, once stretched by a new idea, never regains its original dimensions." The authors of this book went on to write, by way of introduction, "We love books, and we bet you do too. We especially love books that inspire, heal, and transform lives." And later, these words, "We've all found that life becomes richer when we're reading a great book. You go to sleep at night feeling that your time on earth is more valuable, your experience here more worthwhile. You wake up seeing yourself, other people, and the world differently. This is real magic…"

Noted author Deepak Chopra once said that reading has a special transformational power because "it gives you the opportunity to pause and reflect." The authors alluded to earlier write: "When you hold a book in your hands, you're in charge of the pace at which you read and the images you choose to form. You can stop and digest concepts and try on different perceptions and feelings." These minutes or hours can change your life!

One has only to walk into a Barnes and Noble or Border Bookstore to become engaged in the world of books. There are so many. This is not to disparage smaller booksellers. It is to say, however, that we live in a "book-filled world" filled with changing values. We only have to open them up. The books of the ages are contained in our public libraries, and the above-mentioned booksellers remind us of the publishing madness that exists today in our country and in our world.

I used to have an office with a window that gave me a view of our community's library. During the day, with the kids in school and I don't think our youth have much time to read non-school related books and they agree with that assumption, I watched our adult population go in and out carrying bags or armfuls of books. Lives were being changed whether they knew it or not.

The point is, life-changing possibilities are not very far away from any one of us. Old books, new books, our own books, other's books—the potential in them could and can rebirth us and send us off in directions we never dreamed were available to us.

I don't know what your interests may be, but a good book is always better for your personal diet than much of the fare that you can get on the television screens that inhabit many of the rooms in your home. Why not give a new book a try? You might be surprised where it might lead you and how it might change you: how it might enlighten and enliven your life, no matter how old you are or where you are!

EIGHTY-FIVE

It Is Important to Reflect upon Your Own Life's Journey!

Our memories, built as they are upon the recollections we can call to mind, are a wonderful archive to research once in a while. I was reminded of that the other day when my reading exposed me to this thought. The writer was speaking of paging through the leaves of a photo album and viewing the pictures not for the first time but for the umpteenth time. The book of pictures was, for him, a chronicle of the life of his family and of his life as well. He suggested that all of us ought to look through the photo albums that occupy our own shelves or are hidden away in our own closets or attics, for they are an assemblage of pictures that systemically note the passage of our own lives, adding, "Search [them] for the people and places you have loved and learned from yourself, and for those moments in the past—many of them half forgotten—through which you glimpsed, however dimly and fleetingly, the sacredness of your own life."

We all have our own book of heroes: people who have played a major role in our development and life. Teachers: what did I learn from each one of them? Why did I learn from them and not from the others? What were the circumstances behind those learning experiences? Friends: what were our experiences, even the ones we didn't tell our parents about? When did I lose sight of them? I wonder where they are now? What did I learn from each one of them? Where and when? Vocational associates: what did I learn from each one of them?

What did they do to further my career? What did I do to help their careers? Where are they now? What are they doing? How did our relationship foster each one of the paths we have taken since those precious moments we shared together? Our old girlfriends? Well, let us not get into that. And let us not forget our parents. Our kids really need to know more about their grandparents. What did they do to help us in the development our lives? What didn't they do that they should have done? What did I do or what should I have done for my kids? Why didn't I do it?

And the list goes on. The point is, each one of us, as we create our own "book of heroes," will have the chance to see how our lives grew, to consider the changes we have made in our lives, and why.

In these, our reflective years, we have some extra time, and we can use that time to impact the lives of our children and grandchildren with memories and assessments that will assist them as they move through their lives. Like it or not, our lives have and will have some significant impact on their lives. Their actions were and are our actions. Their interests were and are our interests. Their words and phrases, they have heard many of them from us. So they need to know why we used them and why they use them.

Frankly, this is an assignment that will take us the rest of our lives to put on paper, but then, it took us all of our lives to fill the archives we are using to research our answers.

Time well spent! Lessons well learned by us and by our bewildering offspring. Let me tell you of one of the experiences that Dicky Warner and I had in the fourth grade…

Eighty-Six

We Have an Eternity to Fulfill Our Visions?

I heard a poem read at a funeral that set me to thinking. It was the work of Edgar A. Guest and was entitled, "Visions." The lady over whom it was read was one who possessed a real vision for her life, a life that was cut short by a cancer that invaded her body and persisted until it had claimed her life.

The poem spoke, as far as I am concerned, of the tact that someone can hold a vision and work at its fulfillment for many years and see it accomplished much later. This is the last stanza of the poem:

> "Oh, never we reach to our fullest height, and never we do our all. We must turn away at the close of the day when the tools from our fingers fall. But it isn't a failure to hold a dream, that never on earth comes true, For the tasks of worth that we miss on earth, Are reserved for our souls to do."

I am not sure what guest had I mind. I think I get it, but you will have to think about it for yourself. Listen again his final words, "For the tasks of worth that we miss on earth are reserved for our souls to do."

Consider the possibility of having a dream late in life and working toward its fulfillment on this side of life's door with the understanding that if we do not complete it, on this side, we have the chance to fulfill it on the other side. Wow! That is some deep thinking.

Does it say to you, as it does to me, that it is never too late to start dreaming: that the possibilities that come to our minds can reach fulfillment even if we pass on in the process of seeing them accomplished? Another stanza, the third, reads like this:

> "Perhaps they sing at their sweetest now, Those poets of yesterday, And have caught the themes of the golden dreams, Which came from the far away. Perhaps the painters on canvas true, Now see with a clearer eye, And paint the things of the visioning that were theirs in the days gone by."

Now I don't know about you, but I find something really challenging in those words. I can still do some of the things that I had hoped to do, even though I might not see them to completion in the sight of those whom I know and love here on earth.

There are a whole host of dreams that my limited abilities and time make impossible to happen. Reality has to be a part of any goals I set and/or dreams that I have in mind. But there are others that have only been a whisper in my mind that are capable, with my abilities and time, to fulfill.

What are the dreams that you have had, all your life long, that you have not yet satisfied? What goals and aspirations have come to mind, even in these very last years of your life that have the possibility of being fulfilled? Think it over. You can have some of those special, satisfying moments now; and if not, who knows, maybe later…

EIGHTY-SEVEN

Make Today the Most Important Day in Your Life!

"You can't see the forest for the trees!" We have all heard it said. What have all said it! I was reminded of these words by John Naisbitt, the author of one of the classic works of the late twentieth century, *Megatrends*.

He writes, in his book *Mind Set*, of being in Panama City at the time when the canal was being handed over to the nation of Panama by the United States. He tells of flying over the land traversed by the canal "an impenetrable rainforest spread for miles…a denseness that made the jungle under us look like a lush green carpet, through which the blue man-made band of the canal was drawn."

Then a few days later, he went on a hike through the rainforest that surrounded the canal. "It was another world with different perspectives and insights but (it) also (gave) proof that you (can) lose the view of the forest if you are entertained by the trees."

He added, "The distinction between details and the big picture cannot always be experienced in such an exuberant way. But the idea stays the same. You cannot see the forest for the trees. If you lose (a sense of distance), fads can easily block your view."

The words reminded me that the life that I have led has often been lived in the fast lane, if you will; not *fast* in the sense of being lived loosely, but *fast* in the sense that I have moved so quickly through it that I didn't always have time to really think a lot of things through before I did or said something. How many of us are caught up in the speed of the moment and do and say things that we might not have said and done if we had had sufficient time to think the situation or conversation through?

One of the blessings of one's latter years, during the retirement years of life number 2 (after your first retirement) or life number 3 (following your third retirement), is that we can think back over our lifetime and see things as they really were and not as we thought they were. Fads dominate so much of our lives. What we eat, what we hear, our politics, our social customs—most of what life is all about is dominated, in those fast-moving years, by what we see and hear as we swiftly run through our adventure. As a result, things are said and done out of a habit or a feeling that, later on, may not appear as appropriate as they seemed at the time.

Now in these later days, with some leisure time on our hands, we can think ourselves through many of those situations and events that became a part of our own personal history; and possibly we can have the opportunity to reconsider those decision-making moments, etc. and think about correcting some of the decisions that we made: miscalculations in judgment, decisional errors. In these moments, we have the chance to allow a fresh breeze to blow through and over our lives as we slowly reflect upon what we did at some of the crossroads that were a part of our living. Maybe we will decide that we need to go back if the time is still available and move in another direction. It might—in fact, it could change the course and conclusion of our lives.

I think we would be amazed at the liberated feelings that might begin to take hold of our lives. Some of us will gradually find a new freedom in our walk and a new spirit in our determinations. All at once, we will begin to see the forest *and* the individual trees that are a part of it, will lose their attractiveness, and maybe their beauty. Who knows what new adventures, what new possibilities, what new relationships will result because of our actions.

Why not take a few minutes, hours, or days and sit down and think back over the years of your life to see what mistakes you made that you still may have time to correct before you pass on? You might find some new and wonderful blessings in the offing.

Eighty-Eight

Remember: We Make Our Habits and Then Our Habits Make Us!

Denis Waitley reminds us that "the principle of exchanging new habits for old are the same. Whoever we are, we make our habits and then our habits make us, and it happens so subtly that we remain unaware that the process is going on. The bindings of our habits are too small to be felt until they become too strong to be broken. Like comfortable beds that are easy to get into but hard to get out of, literally mindless routines master us unless we master them." And so, as I have already suggested, in our quest to meet our hopes and our dreams, we sometimes forget what we have been doing when we have not been striving for success and our well-being. Too often we do not confront our bad habits until we are ready to move on into a new way of life. At this point in our lives we call it "retirement living."

In this regard, unlike in some areas, to beat those bad habits, "Some changes must come from the outside in." When we practice bad habits over a long period of time, they can so engrain themselves in our attitudes, beliefs, and feelings that escape from them seems almost impossible. In such cases, you must exhibit change, do it, and perform it so that everyone, including you, can see it. I faced that face on the practice tee this afternoon at the golf course. A friend did not take long to show me how I have been miss-hitting for a long time and now, "the bad habit" has to be whipped before I can ever get back to whatever was normal.

REFLECTIONS OF A RELUCTANT RETIREE

Waitley again. "This means that no matter what your past, how many times you've failed or been hurt or haven't reached your goals—no matter how long certain habits have controlled you—you can make a permanent turnaround if you change...your routines."

He then offers three rules for change: (1) "No one can change you and you can't change anyone else. You must admit your need, stop denying our problem, and accept responsibility for changing yourself." It sounds like we must enter into a twelve-step program. You know, "My name is Dick, and I have a problem. This is what it is..."; (2) "Habits aren't broken but are replaced by layering new behavior patterns on top of old ones. This usually takes at least a year or two." Beating our discouragements has to be job one!; (3) "A daily routine, adhered to overtime, will become second nature." Practice makes perfect, for good or bad!

Consequently, for the remainder of my lifetime, I will have to be engaged in adhering to a set of disciplines that I have to set before myself and *do* every day. Frankly, I don't think I am up to that, but I will not really know until I try. I *have* tried, but evidently not enough.

Early to bed, early to rise might give me the time to make some significant changes in my life; adjustments that will enable me to live my life in a successful way. I just have to commit myself to doing it! What does the commercial say, "Just do it!" Well, I am trying. How about you? Where are you? Where do you need to go? What do you need to do? Well, get on with it! How are *you* going to become what you want to be and get where you want to go while you still have the time?

EIGHTY-NINE

Maybe We Need to Find a Fresh, New Perspective for Our Lives?

In a contribution to Jack Canfield's and Gary Hendricks's collection of writings, *You've GOT to Read This Book!*, an Australian TV Producer, Rhonda Byrne, directs our attention to a book by William Wattles entitled, *The Science of Getting Rich*. This is what she had to say: "The longest chapter in Wattles's book is on gratitude, and it's also the chapter that had the most impact on me. Wattles writes that gratitude enables us to create more of what we want in our lives. He says you must focus on all of the wonderful things you have in your life and not on the things that you don't have and then practice being grateful for all of those wonderful things."

I am reminded of the question, "Is your glass half empty or half full?" Byrne suggests that she looked at life as a glass half empty. "I didn't spend much energy on the things that were going well. Instead, I focused on my problems: not having enough money, not having enough time, being under stress. After reading Wattles's book, I completely changed my thinking habits."

For example, "In the area of finance, instead of worrying about the money I didn't have, I was grateful for the money that I did have."

How many of us, on the young side of retirement, look at life as being half empty? We are concerned about our income, our possessions, and our family and the dangers that lie in wait for all of them, of us. We are constantly under stress, and our words and actions show it. We fought with our spouse more than we do now, as we live together on the older side of our retirement.

Years ago, when I would be working on my computer and lost something before I was ready to print it, I would ofttimes lose my temper and speak some bad words to my writing machine. This only happened, I should be quick to add, when I was alone and no one could hear my ranting and raving. In the midst of my temper tantrum, I would feel the front paws of our dog, a small white Maltese, on my leg. He seemed to know that something was wrong, even if I didn't, and he wanted me to know that I was not alone; that he was there, and that, in fact, all was really right with my world.

Suddenly my anger would dissipate, and I was soon able to calm myself down and get along with my life. You see, I suddenly realized that I needed to take a fresh look at the situation, and he let me know about it. I had to learn not to take the problems in my life and myself too seriously. I was nowhere near a life-and-death situation. My glass was, in fact, just half empty at the moment. I needed to realize that that was all right; that I had all that I needed at the present time. Soon I realized my glass was, in fact, half full!

Today, in these latter years, I don't see life as a glass half empty anymore. Now I see it as being half filled. I still cuss my computer, but I know it is just a problem with my lack of patience. Byrne writes of Wattles's words: "I have come to realize that I am so much more than this little physical body. I have control over everything in my life, and there is a power within me that can create whatever I want. All I have to do is to change how I think and feel, and the whole of my life, in every single area, will change—and that's exactly what I have done. In every single area of life, I decided what I wanted, and that's what I've gotten."

Her conclusion is wonderful: "The joy I have in just being alive and being able to be on this marvelous planet one day after another is incredible."

One of the real joys of my retirement is knowing that I have had a blessed life and that I have the chance to share that blessing with others, near and far. I had to be led to the realization that I have a great deal to be thankful for and that I should be very grateful for it. So do you!

My glass is half full! So is yours, I am sure. So don't worry about the other half. It will fill itself up in due time. Relax and enjoy the life that you have and the opportunities that lie before you.

NINETY

There Is Genius to be Found in Truly Wanting What We Really Need!

"Lord, give me what you have made me to want. I praise and thank you for the desire that you have inspired, perfect what you have begun and grant me what you have made me long for." This was the prayer of an eleventh century priest, Anselm of Canterbury, one of the great thinkers of the Middle Ages.

The suggestion of the prayer is that Anselm believed we have simply allowed our desires to become attached to objects or goals which cannot truly fulfill them. Our need, as far as he was concerned, is to fix our desires upon something that can truly satisfy us.

It is the gist of one of Jesus's famed parables, *The Pearl of Great Price*. You will perhaps remember the story. A merchant woman comes upon a pearl of great value. However, in order to have it, she has to sell everything that she has. Why? Because that pearl represents something which she desires with all her heart, mind, and soul.

Alister McGrath offers us this thought: "The merchant, searching for the pearl is, herself, a parable of the long human search for meaning and significance that life has to offer. It is clear from the story that she already possessed many small pearls. She has surrounded herself with the many special things that she thinks are important to her life. However, she is always on the lookout for something more; for something really special. And when that something comes along, she is gladly willing to sell all that she has acquired in order to take hold of it."

He then adds, "Many of the beliefs and values that we take hold of are like those lesser pearls. They seemed worthwhile, and for a time, they offered fulfillment. Yet deep down we knew that there had to be something better."

I wonder sometimes if the pearl we are searching for is not something on the outside of us at all. Is it possible that the supreme pearl is something that can only be found within us? What was it Saint Augustine said, "God has made us for himself, and we are restless until we find ourselves in him." If the "core" is satisfied, can we not find satisfaction anywhere and everywhere?

Some people are forever on the move. They always have to have others around them; they always have to be doing something; they always need *more* stuff! Frankly, I must admit that I have found supreme satisfaction in the simple things in my life—my family, my home, just doing things like reading and gardening. As I think about it, I don't think that I am searching for anything else. I have to be open to something that might come along and draw my attention, but at the moment, I can imagine what that might be.

Maybe that is because now, in my life, I have very few options left. I am truly retired with little chance of returning to the work-a-day world. I have been truly thrown back on myself. The fact of the matter is, I am content! I am happy! I feel satisfaction at the end of every day! I can truly say, thank you for all that I have, and I really don't need anything more of importance and significance to make my life complete.

I think, that as our years mount up and our options begin to vanish, that we need to ask ourselves at certain intervals, "What is the center of my life? What is really important to me today? What are the most important things in my life today? Can I get along without anything else being added to my treasure?"

It is a conversation that we can have with ourselves. We don't need any more input; we just need to think deeply into ourselves and determine if what we are and what we have is consistent with who we want to be. Why not take some moments, or a whole lot of moments, to think this subject through. You might suddenly find that you are all that you want to be; maybe not all you can be, but at that point in your life when you can stop searching and start being?

Ninety-One

Remember: We're Not Home yet!

I came across a rather interesting story. It speaks of a Christian missionary couple who were returning to this country, following twenty years of service in a foreign land. It had been a very satisfactory and, they thought, successful tour of duty. It so happened that Theodore Roosevelt, the former president, was also traveling on that very same vessel. When they arrived in port in New York City, because the former president was onboard, the crowds on the receiving shore were large and celebratory. However, following Roosevelt's departure from the dock, amid the adulation of his followers and others, the missionaries were left to themselves. No one was present to honor or celebrate their years of service or arrival home.

They stood there alone, thinking about what to do next. Their clothes evidenced their lack of funds, being twenty or more years out of date. They counted the money they had in hand and determined that they could hardly afford even the poorest of hotel rooms.

Upon their arrival in their afforded room, they lamented to one another, wondering why God would allow them to arrive home with no one waiting for them with no words of thanks for their work in the field for over twenty years. Then they heard a voice, and the voice said to them, *You are not home yet!*

Those of us who have worked for many years and had a semblance of success in all that we were called upon to do and did not receive the recognition we thought we deserved at the conclusion of our labors, let alone the pension and financial reserves that we wish we had; don't we feel like that missionary couple? I know many who do. How many people, in the midst of their retirement and in the latter days of their lives, need to hear the voice the missionaries heard? "You're not home yet! You need to keep on keeping on!"

Having heard the voice, do we not need to move on, being thankful for the opportunities we have had and the felt successes we enjoyed to fight another day? To work in other ways to make each of our remaining days, weeks, months, and hopefully, years special in our own sight and in the sight of our Maker?

We are not home yet! Right? But we are moving in that direction, and in the time left and available to us, we have many miles to go and many (opportunities) and promises to keep before we go to sleep.

Bring on tomorrow!

Ninety-Two

The Responsibility of Self-Assessment!

It has been reported that a friend once asked the great artist Michelangelo why he had labored so long and so intently over the intricate details while painting the ceiling of the Sistine Chapel. Details so tiny that one would have never noticed them, rightly or wrongly done. "After all," the friend said, "who will know whether it is perfect or not?"

The artist's response was, "I will!" Here was a man who knew that life is interested in the details. We should also remember and know that!

Most of us, during the course of our lives, are regularly confronted by individuals or situations that help us to assess our work. However, once we enter the phase of life that we call retirement, such assessments are few and far between except perhaps those made by our spouse or our children. Hence, the importance of Michelangelo's response, "I will!"

How we spend our time, how we conduct our lives, how we do and satisfy our immediate tasks and responsibilities—they become *our concern*. We become the judge and jury of our work, of the use of our time and the utilization of our abilities, whatever they may be.

So our daily assessment of our tasks, or our weekly or monthly survey of our judgments and actions of what we did or could have done, of what we said, and could have said—they are very important. If we are going to maintain a life of responsibility, if we are going to continue to satisfy in a responsible and commendable way, every task we perform and every word we say, they should be analyzed and graded as if a supervisor might hold us accountable for them.

Who is responsible for the way we live out our lives? *We are!*

Ninety-Three

Do You Have a Grip on Your Life?

Henri Nouwen, the late but highly regarded Roman Catholic priest, remarked that Christianity is not simply another scheme for the never-ending satisfaction of the self. It goes beyond an ego trip and grows into service to others and the giving up of self, surrendering to God. Then he added, "Christianity offers a journey that is not just sweetness and light, but thundering darkness and doubt, thorns as well as roses, nails as well as doves."

There are so many times in our lives when we don't feel like we have our lives together; times when we doubt not only ourselves, but God too; times when we are ready to throw out the baby with the bath and go in another direction; times when we ever wonder why we ever decided to go in the direction we are going, when to go another way would have been perhaps easier and more satisfying. Then there is that vision of Mother Teresa all over again. As individuals, we are very prone to want to give up on so many of our adventures. Life just doesn't seem to be offering us what we want, or even a bit of it.

One of the difficult things in the long days of January, February, and March is to deal with the distractions that are around us. Then we have only time and sometimes too much of that. If we have established a routine, the danger is that routines will be attacked, and in the state of confusion that follows, we will find ourselves out of sine with life. In those moments, suddenly we will find ourselves floundering, searching for a meaningful life without an awareness of what we ought to be doing to find it.

One day, my internet connection went out, and suddenly several of my personal avenues of pleasure and study became unavailable. It felt like the bottom had fallen out of my day, and since I am technologically challenged, to quote a member of my family, I remained out of sorts until I was able to find someone to help me bring it back online and help me to reestablish my routine and bring order again into my life. I find myself compelled to satisfy certain daily obligations. I need to accomplish them regularly, or I end my day with a sense of incompleteness. It goes back to the need to have and carry out a discipline not only my reading and writing but in my diet and in my other activities as well.

I don't seem to be able to live each day unto itself. They all have to be tied together by one or more of the disciplines that I have developed over the years.

There are days when boredom inflicts itself on my mind; when I wish that I knew where my life was going and how I could once again gain the sense of satisfaction and accomplishment that I had in what Bob Buford calls life number 1. That is the challenge that faces me each and every morning and perhaps every evening as well. Getting a grasp on a life that seems like Jell-O in my hands.

I wonder how many of us have to or ought to take an inventory of ourselves fairly regularly to see what we need to do to do the game of life successfully? The pilot and copilot have a checklist. They go through it to determine if the plane is ready to fly. Maybe we need to have a checklist to go through, every once in a while, to determine whether or not our life is ready for the journey that is ahead of us?

NINETY-FOUR

The Importance of Developing an Attitude of Relaxation!

On the other hand, maybe we don't need to have meaning as far as our lives are concerned. Maybe we have had all the meaning we need. Maybe all we need now is a lack of meaning, the opportunity to just relax and enjoy.

My wife and I were in Florida a while back. We visited an adult playland which the guide described as "Disneyland for adults." Over sixty-five thousand retired adults living together in a retirement community dedicated to just having fun. They dance, they golf and softball, swim, do woodwork—over eleven hundred different activities are available each week, and according to the guide, everyone is having fun, a good time. *Meaning*, as far as they are concerned, has taken a backseat to having fun. Maybe that is what life means to them at this point in time: just having fun! Relaxing! Enjoying!

I think that there are a good many people around today who are tired of thinking serious thoughts. Oh, they watch the stock market and their money but only because they are an important part of their life of having fun. They are resources for living, nothing more and nothing less.

Maybe, and I have been slow to understand this because this is not where I am, they are now ready to enjoy life in a very meaningless, meaningful way. No deadlines! No To Do lists. No necessary responsibilities other than satisfying their latest whim and knowing that there is nothing to feel guilty about.

Many people who have had more responsibilities than they had planned for in their developing years have just had enough. Now they are ready to just have some fun! And there are people who need to know this. They need to have their guilt feelings extinguished by their awareness that they don't owe life anything anymore. In fact, it is life that owes them, and now they are free to collect their reward. And they don't even have to pass goal to get it.

For some of us, at a certain point in time, all that life expects of us is to enjoy having fun, relax, and when we are in the mood, reflect! To feel like this, I know, takes some doing.

We probably have to change locations, find people who reflect the feelings that we are looking for, and relax into their lifestyle. Some of us will never be able to do that, and I feel sorry for us; but many of us can and will do it. Disneyland for adults! Not a bad place to live and play and live out our lives. Frankly, it's not for me; but then, we are all different, and our lives do and will show it.

Where would the appropriate place be to spend the rest of your life? Take a look and then act on your decision. However, you had better think very carefully about it.

Ninety-Five

The Liability of Stuff!

In his writing, *What Was I Thinking*, a Presbyterian minister by the name of Steve Brown tells of his encounter with a young man during the Jesus Movement in the '60s and '70s. Brown was a minister serving a church in suburban Boston when a young man by the name of Jamie appeared. He had a ponytail, always wore jeans, and had a smile that would light up the world. I am sure you get the picture.

He participated in the life of the church for a number of years, but then he decided it was time to leave. He said he felt a call to go to Colorado, and nothing could dissuade him from leaving. Brown writes, "I can close my eyes now and see Jamie walking down the hill from the church with his backpack over his shoulders. I had hugged him and promised to pray for him. I'll never forget what he said. 'You'd like to leave too, wouldn't you?' I allowed that I was a bit envious. 'But, Steve,' he said, 'you can't leave, because you can't get everything you have in a backpack. When you do that, you'll be free.' (Those words were more profound than he ever knew.) When I can get it all—my reputation, my stuff, my needs, my dreams, my heart—in my backpack, then I'll be free. It doesn't fit there now, and that's the reason I'm attracted to the world."

Well, when retirement hits and if we have been faithful in preparing the economic side of our life, then it is possible that we can leave. Our proverbial backpack may be bulging, but at that point in our lives, we will be able to head out in a new direction. The possible fulfillment of new dreams is just over the horizon.

How many times have I read of individuals who, upon retirement, find a new direction to take, a new path to walk, a new vocation to unfurl? It may be a workshop in the basement or garage. It may be in the office of a new developing company; I saw an automobile advertisement making that suggestion. It may be as a volunteer in a community organization; it will be somewhere. A new approach to life, a new way of living in the same old house on the same old street in the same old community. Or we might decide to pack up our belongings and move north, south, east, or west.

"You can't leave, because you can't get everything you have in a backpack." Then the kids are gone, we have a new gold watch on our wrist, we have a pension and even some Social Security money and adequate health insurance, and we can now venture out to change the world in a new way: to change our world, if our spouse will let us—to adopt a new way of life. We can describe it as a new calling, but no matter how we define it, we are free to do something we always wanted to do with no holds barred.

So take the time to look in at yourself. Look out at your world. Think with those who love you and whom you love about tomorrow, and make life happy and fulfilling as you walk along with your bulging backpack, ready to change the world around you.

Ninety-Six

How to Continue to be Successful in Your Life!

In their book, *Success Built to Last*, the authors offer up this thought: "Many things in life don't last, but meaning does." They also include these comments, "The harsh truth is that if you don't love what you are doing, you'll lose to someone who does," and "Making a life is as important as making a living." Then this one: "Successful people come to the conclusion that doing something that matters to them is a dream worth their life."

Finally, they quote venture capitalist Ann Winblad, who wrote, "When you skip the step of realizing what makes you tick, then you're taking the big risk that you've not landed on something upon which you can build success that will last."

Sometimes when we really get involved in life, we can become so entranced in what we are doing that we soon don't know why we are doing it; and the longer we do it, the more lost we become in it. The time which we can spend in reflection and reexamination before we take on and become involved in a new venture will allow us the chance to consider the direction in which we would be moving and, if necessary, allow us to re-chart the course we would be taking.

Frederick Buechner suggests that "God's chief purpose in giving us memory is to enable us to go back in time so that if we didn't play [our] roles right the first time around, we can still have another go at it now." Then he adds this thought, "The sad things that happened long ago will always remain part of who we are, just as the glad and gracious things will too. It is through memory that we are able to reclaim much of our lives that we have long since written off. An act like this can be accomplished almost anywhere along life's way, but it is of supreme importance to rethink the direction of our lives when we find ourselves completing our first life," and are ready to enter into what Bob Buford calls life number 2.

As I have stressed on these pages, there is value to be found in working one's way back to the very beginning of one's vocational adventure to see if what we started out to do has been accomplished when we come to the end of our adventure. Sometimes the answer will be yes. At another time, it will be no! If the *no* word pops up, then we need to go back on our decision trail to see where and when we wandered off course. Maybe at that moment time, before it is too late, we can refocus our sense of direction and reach out and accomplish the initial goal or goals we had set for ourselves in life number 1.

Some of us, however, will find that we are too far along life's road to go back and reconfigure our lives. We will have to wait until we move from one life to another. It is at this point in time that we can rethink what we have done and why we did it. Life number 2 becomes the time when we can think about moving on a dream or aspiration that we had in the long-ago days of our youth. Maybe there is still time for us to find and feel a sense of completion in our lives in this particular area or activity.

I think that there is a certain freedom in that exercise. Likely, we will have achieved success, as far as the world is concerned, in our first enterprise. However, just maybe we will find that we have a bad taste in our mouth or a sense of frustration because what we finished doing did not really have any meaning for us. So the words "Making a life is as important as making a living," can be a song we can sing when life number 2 is about to begin.

Reflect! Take a look at the history of your life. Determine what your idea of life was really all about in the beginning. Did you or have you revised that goal? What can you do today to gain a sense of completion, as far as your life is concerned, no matter what that may mean?

BIBLIOGRAPHY

I have drawn heavily, and quoted often, from the following books:

American Council of Learned Societies, Occasional Papers, No. 65.
Blanchard, Bob and Melinda. *Live What You Love.* New York: Sterling Publishing Company, 2005.
Brown, Barbara Taylor. *Leaving Church.* San Francisco: HarperCollins Publishers, 2006.
Brown, Steve. *What Was I Thinking? Things I've Learned Since I Knew It All.* New York: Simon Schuster, 2006.
Buechner, Frederick. *Secrets in The Dark.* San Francisco: HarperCollins Publishers, 2006.
Buechner, Frederick. Listening to Your Life. New York. HarperCollins Publishers, 1992.
Briscoe, Stuart. *Genuine People: Living and Relating As Real Christians.* Wheaton, Illinois: Harold Shaw Publishers, 1988.
*Buford, Bob. *Finishing Well.*
Burkhart, Roy A. *If it Were Not So.* Columbus, Ohio: Community Books.
Canfield, Jack and Hendricks, Gay. *You've GOT to Read This Book! 55 People Tell The Story of the Book That Changed Their Life.* New York: HarperCollins Publishers, 2006.
Danforth, John. *Faith and Politics: How the "moral Values" Debate Divides America and how to Move Forward Together.* New York: Viking/Penguin Group, 2006.
Ervine, St. John G. *The Ship.* New York: Macmillan Publishers, 1922.
Ford, Debbie. *The Best Year of Your Life.* San Francisco: HarperCollins Publishers, 2005

Grumbach, Doris. *The Presence of Absence: On Prayers and an Epiphany*. Boston: Beacon Press, 1998

*Guest, Edgar. George Matthew Adams Service, New York.

Hybels, Bill. *Holy Discontent*. Grand Rapids, Michigan: Zondervan, 2007.

Kazantzakis, Nikos. *Report to Greco*. Simon & Schuster, 1965.

Kidd, Sue Monk. *When the Heart Waits*. San Francisco: HarperCollins Publishers.

Kouzes, James M. and Posner, Barry Z. *A Leader's Legacy*. San Francisco: Jossey-Bass/A Wiley Imprint, 2006.

Kushner, Harold O. *Overcoming Life's Disappointments*. New York: Alfred A. Knopf, 2006.

L'Amour, Louis. *Education of a Wandering Man*. New York: Bantam Books, 1989.

Lamott, Anne. *Plan B! Further Thoughts on Faith*. New York: The Berkeley Publishing Group. Penguin Group, 2005.

Levoy, Gregg. *Callings: Finding and Following an Authentic Life*. New York: Three Rivers Press, 1997

*Leas, Speed B. Creative Leadership Series.

Livingston, Gordon. *Too Soon Old, Too Late Smart*. New York: Marlow & Company/Avalon Publishing, 2004.

McGrath, Alister. *The Unknown God: Searching for Spiritual Fulfilment*. Grand Rapids, Michigan: William B. Eerdmans Publishing Company, 1999.

*Moore, James W. *There's A Hole in Your Soul That Only God Can Fill*. Nashville, Tennessee: Abingdon Press, 2005.

*More, Thomas. *The Soul's Religion: Cultivating a Profoundly Spiritual Way of Life*.

Naisbitt, John. *Mind Set!*. New York: HarperCollins Publishers, 2006.

O'Laughlin, Michael. *God's Beloved: A Spiritual Biography of Henri Nouwen*. Maryknoll, New York: Obis Books, 2004.

Porras, Jerry I., Emery, Stewart, and Thompson, Mark. *Success Built to Last*. New Jersey: Wharton School Pub, 2007.

Peck, M. Scott. *The Road Less Traveled*. New York: Simon & Shuster, 1978.

Peterson, Eugene. *Eat This Book: A Conversation in the Art of Spiritual Reading*. Grand Rapids, Michigan: William B. Eerdmans Publishing Company, 2006.

Piper, John. *Desiring God*. Sisters, Oregon. Multnomah Books, 1986.

Progoff, Ira. *At A Journal Workshop: Revised*. Dialogue House, 1992.

Sanborn, Mark. *The Fred Factor*. Crown Publishing Group, 2004.

Schmidt, Gary. *Spring: A Spiritual Biography of The Seasons*. Jewish Lights Publishing, 2006.

*Simmons, Philip.

Stoddard, Alexandra. *You Are Your Choices: 50 Ways to Live a Good Life*. New York: HarperCollins Publishers, 2007.

Trafford, Abigail. *My Time: Making the Most of the Bonus Decades After Fifty*. Nashville: Upper Room Books, 2006.

*Vaillant, George Eman. *Aging Well*.

*Yancey, Phillip. Prayer.

Waitley, Denis. *Empires of the Mind*. New York: William M. Morrow, Inc., 1995.

Wakefield, Daniel. *Spiritually Incorrect: Finding God in All the Wrong Places*. Woodstock, Vermont: SkyLight Paths. Long Hill Partners, 2004.

Willard, Dallas. The Divine Conspiracy: Rediscovering Our Hidden Life in God. San Francisco: HarperCollins Publishers, 1998.

Wright, N.T. *Simply Christian*. San Francisco: HarperCollins Publishers, 2006.

About the Author

Richard G. Riedel served in the preaching ministry of the Presbyterian Church for over fifty years. He and his wife, Mary Jane, live in Scottsdale, Arizona. They have three grown children and six grandchildren.

CPSIA information can be obtained
at www.ICGtesting.com
Printed in the USA
LVHW042112260422
717237LV00005B/263